BETTER HEALTH

and the

REVERSE EFFECT

by

WALTER A. HEIBY

This is a sampler consisting of material from the **BIG** book *The Reverse Effect: How Vitamins and Minerals Promote Health and CAUSE Disease* by Walter A. Heiby. In addition to acting as an introduction to the *reverse effect,* it is designed to aid scientists in formulating protocols for proposed studies.

MediScience Publishers, P.O. Box 256-P, Deerfield, IL   60015

"Yes, it is crazy, but it is not crazy enough!"
—Niels Bohr. Said to Werner Heisenberg, creator of quantum mechanics and of the *uncertainty principle* and, like Bohr, a Nobel Laureate. Quoted by Gerard Piel in *Science* (Jan. 17, 1986) 231: 201.

Furthermore, Niels, our intelligence keeps us from making it crazy enough!
—Walter A. Heiby

If This Book Is Yours—Mark It Up!

A book becomes truly yours when you mark it up and list key page numbers at either the front or the rear for later review. Mark up this book unless, of course, you have borrowed it from a friend or from the library in which case turn to page 103 and order your personal copy.

Library of Congress Cataloging-in-Publication Data

Heiby, Walter A.
    Better health and the reverse effect.

    "This is a sampler of the big book: The reverse effect: how vitamins and minerals promote health and cause disease by Walter A. Heiby and consists of the opening pages of that book."
    Bibliography: p.
    1. Vitamins in human nutrition. 2. Minerals in human nutrition. I. Heiby, Walter A. The reverse effect. II. Title. [DNLM: 1. Disease--etiology. 2. Health Promotion. 3. Minerals. 4. Vitamins. QU 160 H465b]
QP771.H445 1988   613.2'8   87-12218
ISBN 0-938869-03-5

"It is quite possible to misinterpret what appear to be obvious, easily-explained facts. Listen carefully and you can hear the words of an archaeologist of 100,000 A.D., who is excavating the Vatican. Across the millennia, our time machine brings us the words: 'This was obviously an art school.'"
— Walter A. Heiby, *The New Dynamic Synthesis* (Chicago: The Institute of Dynamic Synthesis, 1967)

"He who knows only his side of the case, knows little of that."
—John Stuart Mill

A *Reverse Effect* . . . . HIV (the AIDS virus) May Cause Immunodeficiency or Immunostimulation

As this book neared completion, John J. Wright et al. published a study in the *New England Journal of Medicine* (Dec. 10, 1987) 317, no. 24: 1516-1520 that suggests HIV may be able to act as a cure for the primary problem it often causes, i.e., immune deficiency. They reported on a single case of a 36-year-old bisexual man who had received a diagnosis of common variable hypogammaglobulinemia in 1974. During the subsequent five years the patient suffered many types of infections and the diagnosis of hypogammaglobulinemia was reconfirmed, in 1979, at the National Institutes of Health. He was found to be seropositive for HIV in 1982 but not in 1981. At least one of his sexual contacts during the early 1980's died of AIDS. For the past two years he has been healthy without evidence of complications associated with either hypogammaglobulinemia or HIV infection. Thus HIV may be able to show a *reverse effect* by working to cause either immunodeficiency or immunostimulation.

IV

"There often is darkness at the foot of a lighthouse."
—Old Spanish proverb

"Wise men argue causes; fools decide them."
—Anacharsis (c. 600 B.C.)

A scientific concept is valuable not to the extent it is
true but to the extent it is fruitful in leading to new ideas.
—Walter A. Heiby

Markers and Underlying Causes

Distinguishing between markers and underlying causes is not
sufficiently recognized as a problem of various sciences.
Cholesterol (an essential chemical required for metabolic
processes), for example, may be merely a marker, rather than
a cause, of cardiovascular disease. If true, reducing
cholesterol would have little bearing on cardiovascular health.
Cholesterol could be the body's patching material to correct
for free-radical damage. If so, our objective should be to
reduce free-radical damage instead of just working to reduce
the mere marker of that damage. Let's concern ourselves with
causes, rather than just with markers, of physiological
problems.

The Rising Price of Science Books

Each year, *Science* reports the average per page price
of books in the natural sciences reviewed during the
previous year. During 1987 (as reported on page 81
of the Jan. 1, 1988 issue) the average per page price
was 12.5¢. At this rate, an 800-page book would
cost about $100.00 and one of 1200 pages about
$150. The current cost of scientific journals is also
astonishing. The price of an annual subscription to
Brain Research is now $3826.00 and that of *Chemical
Abstracts* $8400.00. (Constance Holden, *Science*
[May 22, 1987] 236: 908-909). Regrettably, few
individuals and few libraries can afford this price of
education.

"Progress is the result of some
person's discontent put into
action. Things as they are are
never the best."
— Walter A. Heiby, *Live Your Life*
(New York: Harper and Row,
1964) p. 51.

The Author and the
Reverse Effect

Walter A. Heiby is the instructor of literature research seminars in medicine, dentistry, and nutrition convened at the University of Illinois under the auspices of the *Nutrition for Optimal Health Association*. This has proved to be the ideal setting for development of his *theory of the reverse effect*.

The *theory of the reverse effect* states that there is a good probability that the activity of any substance that is health-promoting or health-destructive in a given concentration may reverse its role and become respectively health-destructive or health-promoting at a different concentration. The author presents numerous examples of vitamins and minerals that reverse their customary action at different concentrations. He speculates that the *reverse effect* may be used to our advantage in finding new therapies for cancer and other diseases. Both *The Reverse Effect: How Vitamins and Minerals Promote Health and CAUSE Disease* and the introductory sampler *Better Health and the Reverse Effect* are replete with creative speculations—new ways of looking at nutritional and medical phenomena.

Now, in the big 1216-page volume, the wealth of research support for the theory is being made available to scientists, physicians, nurses, dietitians, nutritionists and intelligent laymen. Its list of 4821 references is believed to be a record number for a single-author book.[*]

---

[*] The single-author book with the greatest reference density (references per page) is believed to be *Hormesis with Ionizing Radiation* by T.D. Luckey (Boca Raton, Florida: CRC Press, 1980). It is a 222-page book with 1299 references or 5.85 references/page. (Luckey's book contains 168 pages of text or 7.73 references/text page.)

From the BIG book. (Reference numbers refer to that book):

In Vitro Reverse Effects and *In Vivo* Actions

Many of the pages to come will illustrate *reverse effects* using *in vitro* methods. However, it is difficult to relate *in vitro* results to possible *in vivo* actions. The *in vivo* mileau is almost infinitely complex and variable compared with the relative simplicity of *in vitro* conditions. Furthermore, the *in vivo* concentration of each vitamin, mineral, drug, enzyme, hormone or other body chemical may vary from organ to organ. Vitamin C, for example, concentrates in the adrenal gland and zinc in the prostate. Thus, a certain nutrient might show antioxidant action (as vitamins C and E generally do) in most areas of the body. However, in organs concentrating that nutrient a detrimental pro-oxidant action might occur and I speculate that this could be an initiating cause of disease and of side effects. Lipid peroxidation due to vitamin C might conceivably occur even in an organ that does not concentrate this vitamin but instead accumulates iron. An *in vitro* study by David Blake et al.[229] showed that vitamin C in the presence of iron may cause lipid peroxidation in phospholipid liposomes. Could this phenomenon occur *in vivo* in iron-rich organs? Furthermore, vitamin C can concentrate iron in the liver and spleen (of mice) while having no such effect on the heart.[230]

Future physicians will continually face these difficult therapeutic questions: Is it wise to set the dosage of a nutrient or a drug at a level that will promote beneficial actions in most areas of the body while risking a detrimental *reverse effect* in an organ that concentrates that nutrient or drug? How can I set the dosage level to achieve the desired action in my patient while minimizing the risk of side effects caused by a *reverse effect* in a concentrating organ? Much research for generations to come will be required to correlate *in vitro reverse effects* with estimates, organ by organ, of the probable *in vivo* actions of various nutrients and drugs. In the more distant future, *reverse effects* will be controlled by sending nutrients and drugs to specific organs, thereby reducing their entrance into organs in which *reverse effects* might occur. Directed delivery of nutrients and drugs will be achieved by attaching them to carrier molecules with a chemical bond that will be broken only by enzymes in the target organ.

Our life purpose should be to change for the better ourselves and the world.
—Walter A. Heiby

Table of Contents

The importance of controlling stress in animal studies • Factors scientists sometimes improperly ignore

Doctrine of sufficient challenge • Amative individuality • *Reverse effects* common but unrecognized • Small dosages sometimes more dangerous than large ones • The *reverse effect* as a new therapeutic paradigm • Pleasure and a substance's physiological effect • Recommended Dietary Allowances

From page XVIII of the BIG book. Page numbers refer to the BIG book. (Frankly, in reproducing this page we are attempting to entice you to read the BIG book.)

Are You an Index Reader?

Relatively few persons are avid index readers. To most, the suggestion that one read an index straight through from A to Z will seem equivalent to the idea of reading the telephone directory from cover to cover. Index reading, nevertheless, can point out subtleties of a book that may not be found readily with an attentive reading or even several re-readings. A thorough reading of a good index may result in a better learning experience than that provided by a cursory perusal of the book itself.

Right after finishing the Preface of this book, you might like to turn to the Subject Index (which starts on page 1077) for what could be an interesting experience. You may desire to look especially at the large number of subentries under *Reverse effects*. Physicians and medically-oriented scientists may be interested in noting that drug-related *reverse effects* are indexed under *Drugs*. (I view this listing, along with the concepts, theories and speculations on pages 73-74, 164, 260, 326, 786 and 868, as the start of a book someone will write, perhaps entitled *The Reverse Effect in Medicine*. Physicians know much about side effects—little, generally, about *reverse effects*.) A careful reading of the index may suggest the possible existence of *reverse effects* that have not yet been demonstrated. For example, the index shows that on page 752 there is a suggestion selenium may exacerbate arthritis while on page 755 is an indication that selenium may *alleviate* arthritis. Large dosages are often more dangerous than small ones. You may, however, find it intriguing to look in the index under "Dosage" to find examples of large dosages that may be safer than small ones.

Possibly you'll want to check the entries under *Circadian rhythms* for the daily variations in body concentrations of various nutrients. Reading the index will yield such possibly-intriguing entries as the dangers not only of vitamins and minerals but also the dangers of fiber, exercise, peanut butter and water. Readers of the index also will be presented with such possibly-curious entries as the benefits of smoking, caffeine, sugar, obesity and hypertension. Will this be the day you become a confirmed and avid index reader?

"I always had the feeling that the surgeons should have read one more book."
— President John F. Kennedy (in regard to the recurrent problems with his back). Quoted by Kenneth S. Warren, *Coping with the Biomedical Literature* (New York: Praeger Publishers, 1981), p. 18

"Scientific revolutions are very interesting. The way they happen is that most people deny them and resist them. And then there's more and more of an explosion; and there's a paradigm shift."
— Candace Pert, *Science 85* (November, 1985) 6, no. 9: 96

A Preface to be Read

Over the past 15 years I have uncovered a massive amount of information vital to health and longevity. Many of the facts I have discovered are virtually unknown to the public whether they are laymen, medical doctors, dieticians or nutritionists. Much of the information has remained hidden even from scientists themselves except, of course, for the material that relates to their respective specialties. The facts presented in this book were turned up through intensive study of tens of thousands of articles from scientific journals published throughout the world. The monumental project of finding the key material was made possible by doing both manual and computer searches involving *Index Medicus, Biological Abstracts, Chemical Abstracts, Excerpta Medica,* the *Toxicology Data Bank of the Oak*

Ridge National Laboratory, and *Citation Abstracts.*[*]   The task I set for myself was the deciphering of this huge number of technical studies into language understandable by nonspecialists whether they are scientists, dieticians, nutritionists, medical doctors or intelligent laymen.

I hope this book will help you—whether you are a doctor, a scientist, a dietician, a nutritionist or a layman—to learn how to sort out mere popular notions about health from those ideas that are supported by clinical or laboratory evidence. After reading this book—and especially the final chapter—I think you will have a better concept of how information is sometimes managed for profit. Furthermore, it is likely you will by then have increased your ability to not only detect such managed information, but to discover when the popular media are merely acting as progenitors of nutritional nonsense.

Some of the things you are about to learn will shock you. Can the time of day one takes mineral supplements be a factor in health and sexuality (Chapter 7)? Is it possible that vitamin C *causes* cancer (Chapter 6)? What recent research suggests that vitamin D might help *cure* cancer (Chapter 4)? Could it be that vitamin E, widely recommended to make men more potent, may actually cause degeneration of the sex organs (Chapter 2)? Is it possible that the vitamin B complex could *reduce* one's energy level (Chapter 5)? When is vitamin A effective in preventing breast cancer induced in animals by carcinogens and when does it show a *reverse effect* by increasing mammary carcinomas (Chapter 4)? Under what circumstances will zinc work to suppress immunity and when will it strengthen the immune system (Chapter 7)? Instead of being a cancer cure, is it possible that laetrile might be carcinogenic (Chapter 5)? Can it be that lead, a poison in large amounts, is essential for growth in small amounts (Chapter 8)? Could strenuous exercise be a cause of cancer and reduced longevity

---

[*] *Citation Abstracts* (available in libraries of the health sciences) makes it possible to follow up on any given study (including the 4,821 references cited in this book) as future researchers cite these earlier studies. One of the great treasures of a study is likely to be its list of references. The references cited in those references may, in turn, be consulted and so *ad infinitum.* Thus, an endless chain reaction of ever-increasing knowledge can proceed backward in time just as *Citation Abstracts* permits an endless chain reaction perusal of future research relevant to your chosen topic.

(Chapter 10)? Can chemicals called antioxidants—including the much-maligned BHT—give us better health and increased longevity (Chapter 9)?

In addition to presenting new research findings throughout the book, I have developed some of my own health-related hypotheses. My proposed *theory of the reverse effect* may make it possible, via "armchair chemistry" to predict which substances may be therapeutically useful for treating cancer and other diseases. The *reverse effect* may, however, be masked by the very way in which science is so often performed with experimental parameters that have been set too narrowly, along with an improper use of extrapolation. It is sometimes argued that extrapolation is a valid procedure when there exists a theory regarding the functional relationship between variables. I argue, on the contrary, that the theory may be false and that data should be gathered covering wide parameters. In this way it becomes possible not only to prove or to disprove any existing theory, but to allow for the possibility of a new discovery.

Suppose a set of experimental data involving the varying concentrations of a test substance (shown on the X-axis) and the values of a dependent physiological variable (shown on the Y-axis) is properly graphed in this way:

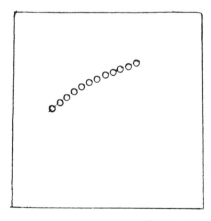

Often a scientist will improperly extrapolate and will presume that the function would graph as follows:

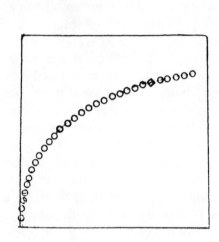

Reality might involve, unknown to the scientist, a *reverse effect* at lower concentrations of the test substance:

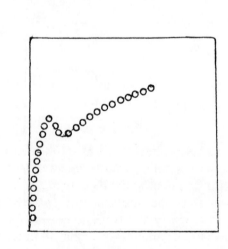

Or, a *reverse effect* might exist at the upper end of the data:

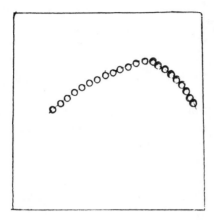

Or, a *reverse effect* might be present at each end:

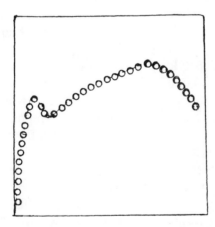

Since, in this example, three reversals exist (two peaks and one trough), we have what I call a *triphasic reverse effect* . (Without the last turn downward the effect would be *biphasic*.) It is possible that at higher concentrations of the substance being tested there could be a fourth reversal to exemplify a *polyphasic reverse effect*. A scientist should extend the parameters of his experiment in order to discover, rather than to hide, new phenomena exemplified by *reverse effects.* Throughout this book we will be examining *reverse effects* of vitamins and minerals as well as, in a few cases, those involving drugs, exercise, x-ray phenomena, etc.

I have referenced virtually every statement unless it is clearly indicated to be my own idea or is a fact or opinion that is widely held. My information is in many cases so unbelievable that I want you to not only question my facts, but I want you to be able to easily check their validity. The citations make it possible for you to ask your local librarian to order for you photostatic copies of the relevant research material. Then you can read the original studies for yourself and come to your own conclusions.

All of us tend to be tree-minded, ignoring the vast forest that lies beyond our immediate perceptions of reality. Some will find in this book merely a few new trees of knowledge about health and longevity. The rare person will use this book as a guide to comprehending the forest of health and longevity perceptions that extends to infinity in all directions. For some, this book may help foster a healthy skepticism in the midst of the noise of nutritional evangelists bent on fostering their own polarized views. But remember, skepticism is healthy only if it allows for the possibility of truth emerging from each of many opposing positions. Truth is always *quasi,* never *absolute.*

Many of the nutritional suggestions that follow will be based on animal experiments and in drawing conclusions for human applications we will sometimes feel less than completely confident. However, we can't wait for everything in nutrition to be proved conclusively. (Of course, nothing ever is.) Those of us with just one life to live are willing to proceed on the basis of probability.

Mankind faces no more intriguing problem than that of how to improve health and increase longevity. I hope you will be as enthralled as I am with the answers now coming from the research centers of contemporary science.

"If we would have new knowledge, we must get us a whole world of new questions."
— Susanne K. Langer, *Philosophy in a New Key* (Cambridge: Harvard University Press, 1948)

Introduction

How to Read Biomedical Literature

I want to encourage you, as you read this book, to ask your librarian to obtain for you photostatic copies of interesting references. Remember, a study that questions the validity of one of your own firmly held opinions may be especially rewarding.

Take cognizance of the fact that prospective studies (ones involving future developments, e.g., after administering a given nutrient) are more apt to lead to reliable conclusions than are retrospective ones (where conclusions are drawn based on past, thus uncontrolled, events). Epidemiological studies may offer reliable suggestions but conclusions drawn from them may not be applicable to individuals who have health parameters greatly deviating from mean values.

When reading a journal article, note whether the purposes of the study are clearly defined. Is it apparent what hypothesis is to be tested or what question is to be answered? In reading the study, be wary of confused writing that should have been corrected by the scientist's editor. If the investigator writes that he fed each mouse 10 mg./kg., does he mean he fed the animal 10 mg. of the test substance per kg. of chow or per kg. of body weight? I think one is proper in downgrading the importance of studies containing unresolved confusion. Is the experimental protocol given in detail? In analyzing the scientific literature, one must especially be on guard against the possibility that the protocol of a study itself may lead to doubtful conclusions no matter how well the study was otherwise done.

In analyzing a given study, examine its protocol to determine if the experiments were performed in a double-blind, controlled manner. In a controlled experiment neither the scientist who is to interpret the results nor the subjects know whether the test substance or a placebo has been administered. That information is known only to a third party, with the results to be decoded only upon termination of the experiment. In many cases, experimenters believe it is unethical (or at least contrary to the dictates of their own conscience) to withhold a thought-to-be-efficacious therapy to, say, one-half of a test group.[*] Thus, they may administer a test substance to all and then compare the results against their opinion of how patients treated with a standard therapy would have responded. In analyzing such studies we must be aware of the power of patients to help cure themselves when given loving care regardless of the efficacy of whatever is being tested. Furthermore, in such cases the scientist/physician may overoptimistically interpret the power of his new therapy. The results of controlled double-blind experiments are more believable, but even those are subject to possible defects in the manner in which they are conducted.

In many cases the results of a triply-blind experiment, as discussed by Adolph Grünbaum,[1a] may be even more reliable than results of one that is double-blind. In a triply-blind experiment the patients are unaware of the group to which they have been assigned, the dispensers do not know what they are administering and those assessing the outcome do not know which were the patients and which were the controls. In some cases, e.g., surgery or psychotherapy, the dispenser cannot be blind and so, at best, we have a double-blind study. (By the way, the cited reference 1a

---

[*] Peter McCullagh[1] quotes the Helsinki Code, which states that "Concern for the interests of the subject must always prevail over the interests of science and society." (Paragraph I.5) Furthermore, this Code also states, "In any medical study every patient—including those of a control group, if any—should be assured of the best proven diagnostic and therapeutic method." (Paragraph II.3)

contains a very valuable discussion of the placebo concept. You may want to request this article from your local library.)

When analyzing an experiment involving human subjects, see if the protocol clearly discloses how they were selected and try to form an opinion whether such selection was valid in terms of the experiment's objectives. Note also how the dropouts were handled. Be wary of the scientist's conclusions if he simply excluded them from his analysis or (far worse) added them to his control group. Keep in mind that many variables (e.g., blood pressure or cholesterol level) will fluctuate over time and the extreme values will tend to regress to the mean values.[1b] Especially low values will tend to rise, and particularly high values will tend to fall, quite irrespective of any given therapy being tested, because of the undue influence of random variation. Such values, if remeasured, are likely to be closer to the mean, a phenomenon called "regression toward the mean."

There are many other considerations in analyzing the appropriateness of an experiment's design. Philip W. Lavori et al.,[2] in discussing prognostic factors other than the treatment itself, says, "If patients who are assigned to separate treatment groups differ before treatment in factors that affect prognosis, such as age, extent of disease or concurrent medical problems, the observed results may be affected by this difference as well as by treatment." Such factors are called "confounding variables," "prognostic factors" or "covariates" and they must be considered or the assessment of the value of the treatment will be biased. Lavori points out that randomization reduces the effects of confounding variables. He says: "Randomization confers several benefits on a study. It protects the rules for treatment assignment from conscious or unconscious manipulation by investigators or patients. Randomization may include the various forms of 'blindness,' but it always ensures that the assignment to treatment groups is left to an objective and indifferent procedure that cannot be predicted. Randomization is not the only way to achieve such protection, but it is the simplest and best understood way to certify that one has done so."

Randomization, however, never provides complete protection, as Thomas A. Louis[3] observes, "against the possibility of producing a trial with unacceptable balance." Louis[3] says, regarding randomization: "Statistical theory tells us that we can expect balance on the average, but provides no iron-clad guarantees for any particular trial. It also tells us that if we check for imbalance on enough covariates (risk factors), we will find some that are significantly out of balance, even if 'perfect' randomization were used." In considering the design and interpretation of studies, John C. Bailer, et al,[4] make the point that "in the absence of a well-defined sampling plan or other support for inference, a finding of 'statistical significance' may be misleading or impossible to interpret, whereas a finding 'not statistically significant' may be meaningless." Valuable suggestions regarding experimental design, appropriateness of subjects and statistical concepts—along with an excellent list of references—will be found in an article by Louis[3] entitled "Critical Issues in the Conduct and Interpretation of Clinical Trials" and in a recent review by Lincoln E. Moses.[5]

Sometimes a purely methodological procedure can be of far greater importance than the experimenter might imagine. Plaut tells about an experiment of S. A. Barnett and J. Burn,[6] who clipped the ears of pups in a rat litter in order to identify the animals. They found that the mothers treated the clipped and unclipped pups differently, thus affecting the results of their study. If they had not been especially alert, a false conclusion based on a defective protocol could have resulted.

The reader of scientific literature must be aware of the possibility that a scientist may not always be studying what he thinks he is studying. If research involves, for example, human intake of high- vs. low-fiber foods, is it possible that the results may have been influenced by the additional milk or cream taken with the bran cereal or by the increased butter used with the bread? Suppose a study is being made of the effects of drinking coffee. Coffee drinkers tend to do more smoking than noncoffee drinkers. Unless the effect of this confounding variable is appreciated and smokers excluded from the study, caffeine could get the blame which might more properly be ascribed to nicotine.

In animal experiments, especially, there may often be little if any appreciation for how the central nervous system can modulate body processes. In particular, Robert Ader[7] points out that it is not a universally accepted premise, even among behavioral scientists, that the central nervous system and immune functions are interrelated.* Without such an appreciation, is a scientist apt to adequately insure that the psychological problems of his animals are not affecting their immune responses in addition to any possible effect of the substance he is testing? Marvin Stein et al.[8] showed that hypothalamic lesions have a significant effect on the immune processes of animals. Nicholas Pavlidis and Michael Chirigos[9] reported that stress inhibited the ability of macrophages to kill tumor cells. Jay R. Kaplan et al.,[10] experimenting with monkeys, reported that "psychosocial factors may influence atherogenesis in the absence of elevated serum lipids." R. H. Gisler et al.[11] say,"Animals used for immunological studies should certainly not be exposed to stressful situations before or during experimentation." It is up to us, the readers of scientific literature, to form a judgment as to the appropriateness of the scientist's protocol which will be disclosed in his published study.

To illustrate the point that the ways in which a scientist works with his animals may (perhaps unbeknownst to him) affect his results, let's cite some studies showing the importance of stress:

1. Stanford B. Friedman et al.[12] reported that when adult mice were inoculated with Coxsackie virus and/or given an electric shock, animals died when both inoculum and the shock were administered, but not when either inoculum or shock was given

---

* In the five years since Ader made that comment there have been many relevant articles, an international symposium (under the auspices of the Princess Liliane Cardiology Foundation in Brussels, Belgium, October 27 and 28, 1983) whose proceedings were published as a book,[7a] as well as other books[7b-f] relating to psychoneural effects on immunity. Other recent studies showing how the immune and neuroendocrine systems are interrelated have been published by J. Edwin Blalock[7g] and by Jean L. Marx.[7h]

alone.[*] Experimental conditions do not generally offer, unknown to the scientist, factors that may be as upsetting as an electrical shock, but still they could be serious enough to affect the results.

2. Contrary to the Friedman study above, Benjamin H. Newberry et al.[13] found that severe electrical shock stress applied to rats in which mammary tumors had been chemically induced (by DMBA) caused a significant reduction in tumor count. On the other hand, Lawrence S. Sklar and Hymie Anisman[13a] reported that a single session of inescapable shock resulted in earlier tumor appearance, exaggeration of tumor size and decreased survival time in mice with syngeneic P815 mastocytoma. Escapable shock, however, had no such effects. In fact, Madelon A. Visintainer, et al,[13b] found that while only 27% of rats receiving inescapable shock rejected a transplanted tumor, 63% of rats receiving escapable shock and 54% of rats receiving no shock rejected the tumor. Lack of control over stress, a psychological variable, seems to sometimes reduce tumor rejection and decrease survival. Stress, while often detrimental, can sometimes be beneficial; the point is that stress should be minimized in a nutritional study.

3. Benjamin H. Newberry et al.[14] demonstrated that chronically administered restraint inhibited the development of DMBA-induced rat mammary tumors. It seems that our perception of what is "good" and "bad" stress may need modification.

4. Andrew A. Monjan and Michael I. Collector[15] reported that daily auditory stress applied to mice for varying lengths of time can,

---

[*] Is it possible that human inoculation is less likely to produce negative side effects if it is performed in the absence of a second perturbing influence? Could the scream of another child be such a second perturbational factor? (The tremendous stress that noise can cause in animals will be discussed soon.) A scream may or may not be stressful. Steven Greer [12a] says, however, in regard to stressful events: "It is the individual's appraisal of and response to an event rather than the event per se which is the nub of the matter."

depending on conditions, either suppress or enhance immune response. Malcolm P. Rogers et al.[16] found that noise stress significantly increased the prevalence of arthritis in rats. Marcus M. Jensen and A. F. Rasmussen[17] reported a progressive hypertrophy of the adrenal glands under the influence of daily three-hour exposures to high intensity sound. They also reported that leukopenia (a decreased white blood cell count) existed during the period of sound stress while leukocytosis (an increase in the number of white blood cells) followed the termination of the stress period. In another study, I. S. Chohan et al.[17a] reported that blood coagulation in rats can be affected by continuous exposure to loud noise. Various blood parameters were changed, including the development of significantly prolonged bleeding time. Ernest A. Peterson[18] says that "noise commonly found in the human environment can cause sustained changes in laboratory animals."* He goes on further to state, "...it is reasonably likely that self-generated noise in dog and monkey quarters is sufficiently high to merit abatement measures." If an experiment is conducted in a noisy laboratory, will results be affected? Possibly, but probably the experimenter would innocently avoid commenting on the condition of his lab. (In the interest of space, a scientist is forced to limit description of his protocol, eliminating possibly important factors.)

There is a kind of "noise" that is often ignored by scientists—that of animal communication. When animals are handled, injected or treated in other ways, they may send supersonic signals[19] to their cagemates or to animals in other cages (where perhaps a different experiment is in progress). The increased corticosterone levels that might result could affect the experimental results.

5.   The time at which stress is introduced can have an important bearing on experimental results. We have just noted some effects

---

* The health of humans is also affected by noise. Baird cites a study by P. Rachootin and J. Olsen[18a] showing occupational exposure of women to noise resulted in hormonal disturbances and reduced fertility.

of sound stress. In another study, Marcus M. Jensen and A. F. Rasmussen[19a] reported that susceptibility of mice to intranasally inoculated vesicular stomatitis virus was significantly altered by daily exposure to three-hour periods of high intensity sound. However, animals inoculated before stress were more susceptible, whereas those inoculated after stress were more resistant to the virus than were the controls. Another study showed the importance of the relative time at which surgical stress occurred. A. R. Turnbull et al.,[19b] in studying the effects of cholecystectomy on guinea pigs after a lethal injection of leukemic cells, found that surgery before the injection of the tumor cells *prolonged* mean survival time by 77%. Surgery one day after the tumor dose did not significantly affect survival, but surgery nine days after the injection of the leukemic cells shortened survival time by 35%. In another study, George F. Solomon et al.[19c] found that when mice, after being given an intravenous injection of Newcastle disease virus, were stressed by repeated random electric shocks preceded by a warning buzzer their interferon response was not altered compared to controls. However, when such stress was given five hours prior to virus inoculation, interferon production was significantly enhanced.

6. The laboratory lighting may influence the experimental results, possibly through involvement of the pineal gland.[20] J. F. Spalding et al.[20] report that black and white mice differ markedly in their reactivity to light of different hue. The importance of laboratory lighting as an experimental variable has been reviewed by John Ott.[21] In a given study you may be examining, did the scientist use the same lighting for his experimental group and for his controls, or was one of the groups housed in a different corner of the room where the lighting (and perhaps the temperature and noise level) differed?

7. Earlier, we noted some benefits of stress. Another benefit of stress is shown by the work of James T. Marsh et al.[22] Eleven

monkeys were subjected to avoidance stress for 24 hours. (They learned to press a telegraph key at a steady rate to avoid a shock that would be delivered every 10 seconds if the lever were not pressed.) After the 24-hour period they were inoculated with type I poliovirus. Twelve control monkeys were similarly inoculated. Seven of the eleven stressed animals survived the infection, whereas only one of the control animals survived. Marsh et al. point out that this study contrasts with findings of *reduced* resistance in mice to virus infection if they are subjected to a different kind of stress called "shuttle box stress." The Marsh study also contrasts with observations of increased susceptibility to poliovirus in hamsters and mice given cortisone before inoculation.

8. The stress of a cold temperature may be beneficial or detrimental. Susan R. Burchfield et al.[23] reported that singly housed male and female rats stressed by cold only before receiving an injection of tumor cells developed significantly smaller tumors than an unstressed group. Rats stressed with cold only after injection of tumor cells developed slightly smaller tumors than the unstressed group. Benjamin H. Newberry and Lee Sengbusch[24] cite other studies showing noxious environmental conditions can either facilitate or inhibit tumor development. When studying the protocol of a given study, try to determine if the scientist minimized stress on his animals unless it was his purpose to stress them.

9. Malcolm P. Rogers[25] reported that if rats that had been immunized with type II collagen were exposed to a cat for a ten-minute period four times a day at six-hour intervals, the stress of that exposure abrogated development of arthritis. They cautioned, however, that the stress may have merely delayed onset of arthritis. The study helps remind us, however, that many types of stress may be beneficial and emphasizes the importance of the scientist minimizing stress in his animals to help assure reliable experimental results.

10. Housing conditions under which animals live may present stresses which could affect an experiment. Either isolation or crowding may generate stresses that can affect experimental validity. Male rats housed together, for example, are prone to fighting (which according to H. M. Weiss et al.[26] may not be bad for them since it prevents stress-related pathology, such as ulceration)[*] but, on the other hand, group housing confounds the experiment because the less dominant animals may be unable to participate. George F. Solomon et al.[29] observed that mixed-sex group housing at high male-female ratios increases the severity of adjuvant-induced arthritis in the male rat. Vernon Riley[30] reported that 92% of female mice carrying an oncogenic virus developed mammary tumors under conditions of extreme stress, including crowded housing and other detrimental environmental circumstances, as contrasted with only 7% in a protected environment. Tumors appeared earliest when females were housed with males, when housed in the vicinity of disturbed mice having elevated corticosterone values (presumably due to contagious anxiety) and when exposed to dust, odor, noise and pheromones.[**] Animals housed more than one to a cage may compete for food. The less aggressive ones may get less food and consequently live longer (or less long if starvation results)—thus negating the "experimental results." Mice housed alone are significantly less susceptible to certain parasites but, on the other hand, show depressed immunity to the parasite *Hymenolepis nana*.[8] In some cases, even humans living

---

[*] Fighting between male rats has other consequences. Henry reported that F. H. Bronson and B. E. Eleftheriou[27] have found such fighting for a few minutes each day leads to an increased adrenal content of cortical hormone. B. L. Welch and A. S. Welch[28] showed that five to ten daily five-minute bouts increase brain noradrenaline and adrenaline.

[**] Riley did not report on the longevity of male mice housed with females relative to male mice housed with other males. However, P. Ebbesen and R. Rask-Nielsen,[31] in studying various types of mice, found that "survival time was much shorter in sex-segregated males of all strains than in nonsegregated males, whereas the survival time was long in all groups of females. (Perhaps sexual intercourse is a longevity factor for male, but not for female, mice.) One variety of sex-segregated male mice (DBA-2) developed a progressive normocytic anemia and reticulocytosis.

alone may show benefits. For example, in a study of prison inmates, David A. D'Atri et al.[32] found that those housed in multiple-occupancy dormitories had significantly higher blood pressures than those housed alone. Crowded conditions may be stressful to men or to animals. Friedman and Glasgow[33] cite animal studies showing that fighting (among males under crowded conditions) may have great influences upon resistance through changes involving the pituitary-adrenocortical axis, reproductive organs and other endocrine functions. However, in favor of crowded housing, they point out that, in another study, such conditions increased the resistance of mice to tuberculosis.* Furthermore, yet another study cited by Stanford B. Friedman and Lowell A. Glasgow[33] showed that female mice housed in groups lived significantly longer after inoculation with encephalomyocarditis virus than when housed alone. Earlier, Howard B. Andervont[35] had reported that virgin mice that were isolated into separate cages at 4 and 20 weeks of age developed mammary tumors at an average age of 9.6 months, while those housed 8 to a cage developed such tumors only after an average age of 11.9 months.** About seven years later, O. Muhlbock[36] did a study related to that of Andervont and achieved similar results. LaBarba, writing about this study, cited Muhlbock as reporting that "animals housed in larger groups consume less food and that caloric intake may be of some importance in tumorigensis." Another study, this one by J. L. Barnett et al.,[37] found that individual penning of pigs resulted in a chronic stress response. Similarly, Vernon Riley[38] reported that female mice had greater

---

* The study referred to, one by Ethel Tobach and Hubert Bloch,[34] in which a Tween albumin culture of M_1 tuberculosis strain was injected intravenously into mice, indicates that "males which were crowded before or after injection of bacilli showed less resistance to tuberculosis than the control mice, whereas females which were crowded before or after injection survived longer than the controls." (Tween solvent may introduce problems as discussed in Chapter 2. Disclosing, in the protocol, the fact that Tween solvent was used allows us to speculate that Tween may have exacerbated any effect caused by the T.B. bacilli.)

** Andervont, writing almost a half-century ago, expressed his concern with the protocol of experiments in these words: "The primary purpose for placing this work on record is to show that in studies on the occurrence of mammary tumors in mice the cages of control and of experimental animals must contain equal numbers of mice."

ability to reject a tumor challenge when housed in groups compared to their single-animal-per-cage counterparts. Joseph T. King et al.[38a] showed that male mice housed 2 per cage or 20 per cage also lived significantly longer than those housed alone. Doreen Berman and Barbara E. Rodin[39] reported on an experiment following dorsal rhizotomy in 44 male rats. (They surgically made a unilateral intradural section of dorsal roots.) Each of 10 isolated animals self-mutilated to an extreme degree with 7 cannibalizing the denervated limb. In contrast, only one of 34 that were housed with female rats showed any sign of self-biting. In any experiments such as this one involving chronic pain, housing conditions may have important bearing on the results. G. S. Wiberg and H. C. Grice[40] reported that rats isolated for long periods became nervous and aggressive and developed caudal dermatitis (scaly tail). They also reported that isolated rats had heavier thyroid glands in addition to heavier adrenals, but lighter spleen and thymus glands compared to group-housed animals. Obviously, colony living is not always stressful for the animals. Such living can be stressful, however, if the colony is disturbed. James P. Henry et al.[41] found that if newborns are removed from a socially organized mouse colony, the social order breaks down. There is fighting among the males and the young are lost due to neglect and injury by the females. James P. Henry et al. reported that there was a high incidence of mammary tumors in such socially disorganized colonies.

Mixing sexes of animals within the same vicinity, although housed in separate cages, can, according to Riley,[38] distort immunological parameters and affect growth of tumors. James Rollin Slonaker[42] had reported, even earlier, that "the activity of male rats in cages near a female tended to follow the rhythm of the female activity." E. P. Durrant[43] also found that the activity of males housed near a female "took on a rhythmic variation agreeing in 95 per cent of instances with that of the associated female." It may be necessary, however, for the males to see the females if such increase in activity is to occur. David R. Lamb et al.[44] reported that when adjacent animals were positioned so they could not see each other, the heterosexual odors and sounds did not result in a significant increase in male activity. H. M. Bruce,[45] however, reports that many animal responses are stimulated by pheromones. He states there is "convincing evidence that the notorious aggression between male mice is released by olfactory signals alone." He also cites a study showing that the domestic cat will display estrus behavior if placed in a cage which recently held a male cat unless the cage has been washed.

Housing conditions often provide a confusing element in the attempt to judge an experiment's protocol. However, in making judgments regarding a given study, I think it proper to be suspicious of an experiment performed under extremely crowded conditions. The resulting stresses could negate the conclusions being drawn by the scientist in charge. Nevertheless, it may not be the crowding per se that is negative but simply the resulting physical contact. S. Michael Plaut et al.[46] reported that in studying mice infected with *Plasmodium berghei,* which produces malaria in rodents, cage size did not affect the mortality rate. They concluded that "the housing effect is dependent upon population size, rather than density." The investigators went on to say, "grouped mice separated by screening died as slowly as individuals, suggesting a role of physical contact in the high mortality rate of grouped mice." Chevedoff et al. cite a study by V. Riley and D. Spackman[47] who, "using cage densities from 1 to 20 animals/cage, failed to repeat earlier results in mice in which tumor incidence was found related to cage density. They concluded that crowding per se is not stressful provided that the overall housing environment is not stressful." Earlier, June Marchant[48] concluded one of her own studies by saying: "It is impossible to make any definite statements about the effect of particular social conditions on susceptibility to breast tumor induction by this or that carcinogen. Each genetic type responds in its own way to a particular carcinogen and may respond in a somewhat different way to another carcinogen. Different social conditions with their accompanying hormonal disturbances do not always have the same kind of effects on breast

tumor induction in different genetic types of mice." A study by
Patricia F. Hadaway et al.[49] bears out the importance of housing
considerations if animals self-administer substances. When
morphine-sucrose solutions were self-administered by rats,
isolated females drank 5 times as much as colony rats and isolated
males 16 times as much. The scientists commented: "If this
housing effect proved to be a general phenomenon, it would
suggest that the influence of laboratory conditions per se must be
emphasized more in the interpretation of self-administration
studies." Either excessive crowding or isolation can sometimes
influence the results of an experiment. Experimental animals and
controls must be housed under "identical" conditions. If this has
not been done we should rightfully downgrade the reliability of a
scientist's "results."

11. Were animals "handled" as infants and/or were they handled
during the course of the experiment? George F. Solomon[50]
observes that there are conflicting results regarding handling of
infant rats and their later experience with respect to tumor growth.
He notes that G. Newton et al.[51] found that rats held and stroked
for 10 minutes daily after weaning and implanted with Walker
carcinoma 256 two days after cessation of handling survived
significantly longer and had smaller adrenals than nonhandled
controls. In contrast, Solomon et al. cite the work of S. Levine
and C. Cohen[52] where mice handled for the first 24 days of life
showed shorter survival times after transplantation of leukemia as
adults. Riley[30] found that merely handling mice for tumor
inspection, provides stress that increased tumor production.
Stanford B. Friedman et al.[53] similarly found that simply placing
rats in experimental cages increased their plasma corticosterone
levels. These studies contrast with those of Robert M. Nerem and
Murina J. Levesque,[54] reported in more detail in Chapter 1, that
showed rabbits held, petted, talked to and played with had better
health. Of course, there is a big difference

between "handling" and "petting" and the results of handling may vary with species and with the disease being studied. Solomon et al.,[50] even though they cited studies showing detrimental effects of handling, say: "It seemed possible that one of the chief consequences of infantile stimulation is to endow the organism with the capacity to make fine discriminations concerning the relevant aspects of the environment. This view seems to be supported by evidence that manipulated animals showed less adrenal response to a new situation and quicker habituation." Robert Ader and Stanford B. Friedman[54a] reported that rats handled during the preweaning period showed a reduced rate of tumor development relative to unmanipulated controls. Ader[55] also found that, "among individually housed animals, handling experience during the first 3 weeks of life decreased susceptibility to gastric erosions." He concluded that "early life experiences can modify a genetically determined susceptibility to disease."

12. We have already noted some housing-related effects on hormone levels. Stephen H. Vessey[56] cites many other studies showing the effect of various stressors on the production of adrenocortical hormones. Grouped mice not only had heavier adrenal glands, but lower numbers of circulating eosinophils relative to isolated mice. Rats housed in colonies had higher levels of plasma corticosterone than those housed in groups of four. Another study cited by Vessey showed groups of 20 had higher corticosterone levels than did those housed alone. Interestingly, David E. Davis and John C. Christian[57] found that group-housed male mice ranking low in their social "pecking" order have heavier adrenal glands than high-ranking mice (Figure 1). Davis and Christian concluded that these findings suggest low-ranking mice are subjected to more physical and psychological stressing stimuli. Furthermore, male mice housed in groups have heavier adrenal glands than those kept in isolation. This contrasts, however, with the finding reported by Paul Brain[58] that isolated female rats have relatively smaller adrenal glands than those housed in groups. (Brain also cites many studies

that show isolation increases gonadal activity in males and that isolated males have heavier sex accessories than group-housed rats. Brain notes that this also may be true of female rats.) Brain[58] cites several studies showing that the turnover rate of neurotransmitters in the brain of isolated mice is lower than in those that are group-housed. Friedman and Glasgow[33] speculate that "the adrenocorticosteroids, and probably other hormones, might act either alone or in conjunction with other physiological processes to modify host susceptibility as a result of psychologic stress." They point out that the modified resistance might be due to the known influence of adrenocortical hormones upon antibody levels[59] and interferon production.[60] They quote I. E. Bush[61] as saying: "Our whole concept of the adrenal cortex as a gland the secretions of which regulate an as yet undiscovered metabolic process that affects the metabolism of carbohydrate, protein and other substances is thrown into confusion by the suggestion that the most important natural stimulus to the activity of the gland is psychological stress." Histamine may also be influenced by stress. W. Cassell et al.[61a] reported that mice exposed to a group environment had a high tissue concentration of histamine. This is in line with a finding by B. Jencks[61b] showing that mice reared in groups had larger numbers of subcutaneous mast cells than isolated animals. (Is it possible that a copious histamine response to stress might be an unsuspected influence in studies using vitamin C—a vitamin that destroys histamine?) When analyzing an experiment, ask yourself if the scientist took cognizance of the problem of insuring the psychological health of his subjects (animal or human) by minimizing stressful conditions.

In studying the protocol of an experiment, be cognizant of the possibility that the scientist may have improperly ignored still other factors:

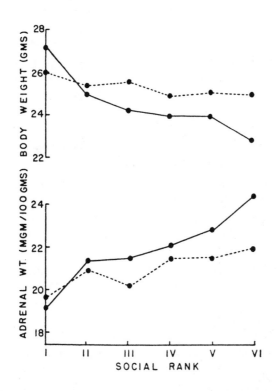

Figure 1. Relation of body weight and rank (upper lines) and adrenal size and rank (lower lines) to social rank in mice. Dotted line refers to weight at start and solid line refers to weight at end of ten days. Reproduced from David E. Davis and John J. Christian, *Proc. of the Society for Experimental Biology and Medicine* (1957) 94: 728-731, with permission. Is it not conceivable that stress might have such an overwhelming influence on adrenal action as to unduly influence a nutritional study? Stress must be controlled if one is to draw valid nutritional conclusions.

1. Did the experimenter take precautions to avoid a conditioned response in his animals that might have affected his results?

Mason tells about a study by F. H. Bronson and B. E. Eleftheriou[62] which showed that merely exposing a subordinate mouse to fighters—especially if the subject mouse has a previous history of defeat in combat—can produce adrenal cortical responses as great as if he had been attacked and defeated. J. W. Mason[63] states that a study he did with J. V. Brady and M. Sidman "showed that a conditioned emotional response, elicited simply by presentation of a mild clicking noise that had been previously paired with electrical shock, was associated with marked plasma 17-hydroxycorticosteroid elevations in the monkey." There are other examples of conditioned responses. Robert Ader and Nicholas Cohen[64] administered to rats the drug cyclophosphamide (the unconditioned stimulus), a substance known to cause immunosuppression. Simultaneously, they gave a distinctly flavored drinking solution of saccharin (the conditioned stimulus), a substance that has no such effect. After training in this manner, the rats were allowed to recover. Then later, when saccharin was given alone, an immunosuppressive effect was produced, illustrating a conditioned response.*

Michael Russell et al.[65] recently showed that histamine, so important in allergic reactions, may be released as a learned response. When an immunologic challenge was paired with the presentation of an odor, guinea pigs showed a plasma histamine response. Later, those guinea pigs showed a plasma histamine response when presented with the odor alone. The experimenters concluded that the study "suggests that the immune response can be enhanced through activity of the central nervous system." Is it possible that, in a study you may be investigating, the animals

---

* More recently, Ader et al.[64a] reported that such conditioning can reduce by 50% the amount of cyclophosphamide needed to control the murine version of the human autoimmune disease lupus erythematosus. Such a finding may eventually lead to human conditioning therapies that might permit similar reductions in drug dosages. Recalling Pavlov and his dogs, need we be limited to using chemicals to potentiate drugs? Could we condition the immune system of a lupus patient to be depressed when given just half of the normal amount of an immune-suppressing drug if that drug were given coincidentally with the ringing of a bell? Could we, on the other hand, condition the immune system of a cancer patient to greater stimulation with an immuno-stimulating drug administered to the sound of a bell?

might have been conditioned to the injection procedure, or to the body odor of the caretaker, or to a certain food, or to the mere opening of their cage doors to react with an increase in plasma corticosteroid regardless of any nutrient or drug the scientist was testing? S. Michael Plaut[66] states, "In many cases, the effects of an early life experience are not apparent until the animal is faced with an appropriate stimulus situation later in life." This suggests that scientists must know their animal supplier and know the precautions he takes for avoiding conditioned responses in his animals. As readers of scientific literature we have to assume the scientists are cognizant of the possibility of such conditioned responses and that they have discussed this problem with their animal supplier. Could it be, however, that laxity in this matter may sometimes be a reason results of different, but similar, experiments are not always the same?

2. We saw earlier that the time at which stress is introduced can greatly affect the results of an experiment. Is it possible that, in a study you may be analyzing, the sequence in which drugs or nutrients were administered or the sequence in which procedures were performed might have influenced the results? Peraino et al.[66a] reported, for example, that phenobarbital administered to rats having liver cancer that was induced by 2-acetylaminofluorene either inhibited or enhanced growth of the cancer, depending on when the phenobarbital was given. If the phenobarbital was given simultaneously with the carcinogen, there was no protective effect; if given after the rats had been exposed to the carcinogen, there was an enhancing effect on tumor incidence.

3. Could one or more circadian rhythms be at work that might influence the experimental results? Ader,[67] studying group-housed rats who were sacrificed sequentially at 90-second intervals, found that "the elevation in plasma corticosterone levels shown by the rats sampled at the crest in the daily cycles is relatively slight as compared to the nearly 5-fold increase in the

corticosterone levels shown by the last animal to be sampled at the trough in the adrenocortical cycle." In another study, Ader [68] reported that rats immobilized at the peak as compared with the trough in the 24-hour activity cycle were more susceptible to gastric erosions. In yet another study, Robert Ader and S. B. Friedman[69] observed that "the time course of the plasma corticosterone response to environmental stimulation depends on the duration of the stimulation and the point in the 24-hour adrenocortical rhythm upon which the stimulation is superimposed." In other research, Alexander H. Friedman and Charles A. Walker[70] reported that histamine levels in the caudate nucleus and midbrain of rats undergo a circadian rhythm and are maximal when body temperature and motor activity are maximal. M. P. Rogers et al.[71] have reported a diurnal variation in natural killer cell activity. If a test substance were to be administered at the time of day when natural killer cell activity was low, would a possible increase in animal death rate be due to that substance or due to the time of day during which it was given? Does the study's protocol consider the possibility that the diurnal variation of plasma coricosterone, of histamine and of natural killer cell activity could be relevant to the experiment being performed?

Friedman et al.[72] point out that sometimes a nutritional deficiency can weaken a microorganism, but sometimes such a deficiency can strengthen other microorganisms (while probably weakening the host).* A scientist, while perhaps taking cognizance of such facts, may improperly ignore the possible chronicity of an infection due to such microorganisms.[73] Studying an experiment's protocol tells us if the scientist in charge is aware of the possible influence of circadian rhythms on his work. Ader[74] cautions that:

---

* Friedman et al.[72] say: "It cannot be predicted whether a specified experimental stimulation will increase, decrease, or not influence host resistance on any a priori grounds. Rather, it has been our view that whether or not a given form of stimulation is detrimental to the host depends upon the particular infectious agent (or disease process) to which the animal is subsequently subjected. Therefore, it seems best to avoid, whenever possible, the very use of the word 'stress,' since it connotes, to many, a deleterious effect on the organism."

The results and interpretation of any study on the effects of the adrenocortical system on conditioned emotional responses (and, perhaps, other conditioned responses) would be determined by the time of day at which different experimenters decided it was convenient to observe their animals. Moreover, unless the light-dark schedule and the time in this schedule were specified, discrepancies between studies would be impossible to evaluate fully. On the basis of these data it does not seem facetious to ask how many discrepancies in the literature are attributable not to who is right and who is wrong but to when the behavior was sampled.

Then, too, the time of day a nutrient or drug is administered may have a great effect on animals, including humans. The science of chronobiology has had its own journal (called *Chronobiologia*) since 1974. Examples of chronobiological effects of potassium, iron, zinc and of other nutrients can be found throughout this book.

4. Was an appropriate animal species used in the study? E. A. Emken[74a] points out that rats have enzyme systems capable of synthesizing many fatty acid isomers which humans may not be able to produce. If so, rat studies in this area might be misleading if extrapolated to man. If it is desired to learn something conceivably applicable to human male sexuality, the rat may be a better experimental animal than the mouse. Morton Rothstein[75] relates that basal levels of testosterone do not decrease with age in mice but do decline in the rat (as in the human male). However, S. Mitchell Harman et al.[75a] reported that the Leydig cells in the testes of aged rats respond to gonadotrophin stimulation far better than do those of aged men. Thus the rat may, as Harman et al. say, "be a poor species in which to attempt to elucidate the nature of age-acquired defects of Leydig cell function."

If an experiment involves use of penicillin with guinea pigs, has the fact, as stated by G. Miescher and C. Böhm,[76] that penicillin is 1000 times more toxic to these animals than to mice been taken into consideration? The cardiac drug digitoxin is toxic at very low levels in the cat, but only at very high levels in the guinea pig. The dosage of oral LD50—at which 50% of the animals will live and 50% will die—is just .18 mg./kg. in the cat, but a much larger 60 mg./kg. in the guinea pig.[76a] Mankind's use of foxglove *(Digitalis purpurea)* that contains this drug goes back hundreds of years so that history was able to guide physicians in establishing therapeutic dosages. If we had relied on the cat or the guinea pig reaction to this drug, we could have been badly misguided.

All scientists know, if they are conducting a vitamin C experiment, the difference between using an animal species that makes vitamin C (such as the rat) and one that does not (such as the guinea pig). But when doing a study involving the effect of honey, does the experimental protocol involve an animal that does not naturally eat honey (such as the rat or mouse) or one that does (such as the bear, sloth bear, ratel or kinkajou)? The ancestors of these latter animals have, like those of contemporary human beings, been eating honey for thousands, perhaps for millions of years, and should therefore be more appropriate experimental subjects.

John B. Jemmott, III et al.[77] have shown that academic stress may affect the immune system of students, as measured by the secretion of salivary immunoglobulin. If the protocol of an experiment discloses the fact that students were used as subjects, were academic pressures considered by the scientist in charge? Students may not be appropriate "animals" for some studies. Other persons under the stress of a large number of life-change events show, as Jemmott, III et al. note, an increased incidence of infectious disease, allergic responses, as well as cardiovascular and psychiatric symptoms. Ziad Kronfol et al.[78] have shown that mood states and immunity may be related. They found defective lymphocyte function in patients with primary depressive illness. (In such studies it is very difficult to separate cause and effect. Did the depression lead to lowered lymphocyte levels, as Kronfol implies, or did the depressed lymphocyte levels lead to depression?) Stanley M. Bierman[79] has developed the concept that recurrent genital herpes may have a psychoneuroimmunologic basis. Similarly, emotional stress factors in the development of multiple sclerosis are discussed by Sharon Warren et al.[80] while psycho-social risk factors in the development of infectious mononucleosis are covered by Stanislav V. Kasl et al.[81] Studies by Richard B. Skekelle et al. [82] and by Cary L. Cooper[83] and by others[84] suggest that psychological depression and other social psychological factors are related to the impairment of mechanisms preventing the establishment and spread of cancer cells. Lawrence E. Hinkle, Jr. et al. [85] make the point, however, that their findings suggest, in regard to the determinants of genetic and environmental illness, the actual life situations encountered are less important than the way in which these situations are perceived. Nevertheless, persons undergoing many life-change events or who are psychologically depressed might be inappropriate subjects for some nutritional studies. Different affective states can be a factor in causing various physiological responses. How carefully does the experiment's protocol minimize such perturbations?

5. Assuming an appropriate animal species has been used, did the experimenter take the necessary precautions to achieve his objective? Many animals are coprophagic—they eat their own feces or the feces of their cagemates. Coprophagic animals normally eat 30 to 50% of their feces.[86] When they are not allowed to engage in this practice, detrimental effects are observed.[86-91] B. K. Armstrong and A. Softly[92] reported that growth was inhibited (as shown in Figure 2) in rats prevented from coprophagy. (Since the animals eat directly from the anus, jackets,[92] collars[92a] or anal caps[92b] must be attached to the animals when it is desired to stop coprophagy.) In consuming feces, the

animals get large amounts of the vitamin B complex, a fact that must be considered in the protocol of an experiment that involves any of these vitamins. If this nutritional source is not controlled, the experimental results may be subject to misinterpretation. Coprophagy can, however, cause animals to develop intestinal infections,[93] and so the experimenter must also be on guard against this eventuality. When you analyze the protocol of any animal experiment involving members of the vitamin B complex, decide whether or not coprophagy might negate the conclusions. On the other hand, if the experimenter restricted coprophagy, did he consider the possibility that in doing so, he may have worsened the condition of his animals?

Another factor in influencing the results of an experiment is the health of the experimental subjects. Vernon Riley et al. [93a] warn that it is essential to the control of inadvertent stress to eliminate the generally unrecognized LDH-virus contamination for experimental mice, tumors and oncogenic virus preparations. Riley and his associates further caution that changes occur in plasma corticosterone levels, the thymus, macrophages, T cells and B cells, as well as in other immunological factors of mice infected with this ubiquitous virus. When the results of a seemingly identical experiment fail to replicate those of an earlier experiment, it may be that sick mice were inadvertently used in one of the studies.*

6. If experiments are being done with chromium, zinc or copper, were wood, galvanized metal, stainless steel or plastic cages used? It seems possible that chromium obtained from gnawing on stainless steel cages might affect nutritional studies involving chromium. Studies regarding zinc may be invalid if the animals received the metal by gnawing on the galvanized metal cage in

---

* It would be inappropriate to consider here the ethics of how animals are treated in the laboratory. Those interested are referred to a recent article, "The Use of Animals in Research," by John K. Inglehart[93b] and another titled "Regulation of Animal Experimentation" by Thomas D. Overcast and Bruce D. Sales.[93c] Entirely apart from ethical considerations, however, when animals are mistreated to the point they become ill, the results of experiments become unreliable.

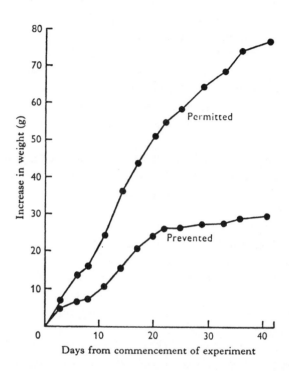

Figure 2. Increase in mean weights over six weeks of rats in whom coprophagy was permitted or prevented on the same diet. Graph reproduced from B. K. Armstrong and A. Softly, *British Jrl. of Nutrition* (1966) 20: 595-598. Reprinted with permission of the publisher, Cambridge University Press. Experiments not considering coprophagy as a nutritional source of the vitamin B complex may be subject to misinterpretation.

addition to the measured amounts received in their diet. For that matter, the zinc received through gnawing on the cage might depress absorption of the dietary copper or selenium that may be factors in the study. Research by Douglas K. Obeck[94] did, in fact, show that four rhesus monkeys and their infants kept in galvanized enclosures had significantly depressed plasma copper

values and significantly elevated plasma zinc and liver zinc
levels. They developed achromotrichia (absence of hair pigment),
alopecia (baldness) and weakness that varied from moderate to
severe, while three infants kept in stainless steel cages were
clinically normal. As we will see in Chapters 3 and 7, zinc is a
factor in prostaglandin metabolism. Some prostaglandin studies
conducted using animals housed in galvanized cages might,
therefore, lead to questionable results.

7. Scientists may sometimes improperly experiment with nutrients,
    such as vitamins and minerals, as if they were unessential.
    Maxine Briggs[94a] points out, in reference to ascorbic acid (AA)
    studies, that:

> Unlike other drugs used against infectious diseases, AA
> is also a nutrient, though being used at nonphysiological
> doses. Nevertheless, in double-blind studies, especially
> where there is no cross-over, it is essential to be certain
> that nutrient intake is adequate in both groups, so that
> high-dose AA is not being used merely to correct a
> deficiency of vitamin C that could have been corrected
> with a much lower dose. Very few of the published
> studies have determined either the dietary vitamin C
> intake of their volunteers, or any laboratory index of
> vitamin C status (such as leukocyte concentrations or 24-
> hour urinary output).

In your study of scientific literature, look at the experiment's
protocol and ask yourself this question: Were adequate steps
taken to assure that the experimental subjects being given a
certain nutrient were not deficient in that nutrient before the
experiment began? If they were deficient before the study began,
simply giving them enough of the nutrient to satisfy the RDA
(Recommended Dietary Allowances of the National Academy of
Sciences) might have produced the same good results that the

experimenter may have attributed to the megadoses he administered.

8. What other factors may have been ignored that might modify the experimental results? (You may never know. Scientists are often lax in disclosing details of an experiment's protocol.) M. W. Fox[95] says:

> Color of clothing most likely has little effect on rats, but the odors of different caretakers may be important. I think cage position is a serious question in rat colonies. If you don't regularly change the cage positions, rats at the top of the rack would have very different experiences from those on the bottom rack. You might note that those on the bottom are under a different light intensity, temperature, and so on; such variables can be controlled by rotation of the cages.*

9. Could the nature of a laboratory animal's diet lead the experimenter to false conclusions regarding the probable human effects of the nutrients or toxins being studied? A. Wise and D. J. Gilburt[95b] noted B. H. Ershoff[95c,d] and D. Kritchevsky [95e] have shown that fiber in the diet of laboratory animals affected the toxicity of many test chemicals. Such effects could conceivably sometimes lead to erroneous conclusions regarding the safety of certain chemicals in the human environment.

Fiber in the human or animal diet is widely considered to be protective against colon cancer. However, as recently as 1986, David M. Klurfeld et al.[95f] cautioned that isolated cellulose, which is the standard fiber source in semipurified diets for biomedical research, may not give results comparable to feeding intact dietary fiber. They found that rats fed a fiber-free diet had a

---

* Friedman and Ader[95a] reported, however, that "merely placing rats in a new environment resulted in a significant rise in corticosterone levels," the magnitude of which "depends upon when during the 24-hour adrenocortical rhythm such stimulation is imposed."

71% incidence of colon cancer after six weekly gavages of the
chemical 1,2-dimethylhydrazine (DMH). On the other hand,
those fed 5%, 10% or 20% powdered or microcrystalline
cellulose for six months following similar gavages of DMH had
colon tumor incidences of, respectively, 75%, 92% and 100%.

Then too, Victor Herbert,[95g] also writing in 1986, cited a
study by L. R. Jacobs[95h] showing that, "A 20 percent wheat bran
dietary supplement increased by more than three times the
numbers of colonic adenomas and adenocarcinomas in rats given
1,2-dimethylhydrazine." Furthermore, Hugh J. Freeman et al.[95i]
reported that when mice were administered 1,2-
dimethylhydrazine, a diet containing 4.5% or 9.0% purified
cellulose was protective against colon cancer (rather opposite to
the results of the Klurfeld group). On the 9% pectin diet, the
number of small bowel tumors was increased. Other studies cited
by Hugh J. Freeman[95j] and done by K. Wakabayashi et al.[95k] and
by K. Watanabe et al.[95l] showed that carrageenan (a
polysaccharide fiber derived from red marine algae that is used in
food as a stabilizing, jelling or viscosity agent) enhanced
chemically-induced colon carcinogenesis and even caused rodent
colon cancer.

Obviously, it is simplistic to categorize various fibers simply
as "fiber." Different fibers consumed under varying
circumstances have diverse effects. To conclude that modest
amounts of fiber in the human diet may be dangerous based on
experiments with animals that had been fed either large amounts
of cellulose or of wheat bran and administered DMH would be
improper, but the questioning attitude that asks "why the
difference" could lead to good discoveries. Many studies
continue to suggest, of course, that fiber used in modest amounts
is protective against colon cancer. For now, our primary concern
is that, when studying the protocol of an experiment involving
animals, we ask ourselves if the diet fed them might have
contained enough fiber to influence the outcome and to affect the
conclusions that were drawn. Furthermore, various fibers
contain different proportions of celluloses, hemicelluloses, pectin

and lignin. Therefore, a conclusion regarding a given fiber at a certain concentration in one animal system must not be presumed valid for another fiber at a different concentration in another human or nonhuman animal system.

10. Much animal research is performed in order to draw conclusions that might benefit the health of humans. However, one must always be cautious about extrapolating animal results to man. In reading scientific papers, observe whether the author made such extrapolations cautiously. Plaut quotes R. A. Hinde[96] as writing, "Apparently close similarities between species may prove to be merely paralleled evolutionary adaptations to a similar environment, and rest on quite different causal bases." Plaut goes on to cite S. A. Barnett[97] who wrote, "Choose the right animal species and you can 'prove' anything you like." Animal diseases are not always similar to the corresponding disease in man. Animal muscular dystrophy is not. Absorption of a given nutrient in an animal may be greater or less than it would be in man. The amount of zinc taken up by the rat and reaching internal organs in five hours was found to be four to six times greater when vitamin C was present.[96a] In humans, however, vitamin C seems to neither enhance nor inhibit the biological availability of orally ingested zinc.[96a] One must be cautious about assuming that a useful nutrient/body weight dosage in an animal is anything more than suggestive of what might be a useful dosage in man.* Furthermore, one must not assume that

---

* In Chapter 1 we will discuss the recommended dietary allowances (RDA) for various nutrients as determined by the National Academy of Sciences. However, requirements for laboratory animals, even if they are primates, may be far different. For example, the National Academy of Sciences[98] recommends that nonhuman primates obtain 10,000-15,000 I.U./kg. of vitamin A from their diet. (Man eats about one kg. of food daily, yet his RDA is only 5,000 units.) The Academy recommends that nonhuman primates receive 2 mg./kg. diet of iodine, 180 mg./kg. diet of iron and 40 mg./kg. diet of manganese. This contrasts with a human RDA of a mere 150 mcg. (1/14 as much) for iodine; 10 mg. for men and 18 mg. for women (1/18 and 1/10 as much respectively) for iron; and 2.5 to 5 mg. (1/16 to 1/8 as much) for manganese. Not only absorption differences but the generally higher metabolic rates in nonhuman primates are factors in the recommendation that laboratory animals receive a higher vitamin and mineral intake than is suggested for humans.

absorption and utilization of a given substance will be the same
for different persons. (A difference in stomach acid concentration
might have a big influence.) Then too, the method of
administering a nutrient or drug has a great bearing on its
effectiveness. In analyzing an experiment, observe whether the
studied substance was administered orally, by injection,
sublingually (under the tongue), buccally (through the buccal
glands in the cheeks), rectally or nasally. Usually, injection of a
given substance will, for example, be far more potent than if the
same amount were administered orally. Generally, oral
administration puts the least amount of nutrient or drug into the
body since the substance has to not only contend with the often
destructive action of the gastric and pancreatic juices, but then
has to find its way past the brush border into the body proper.
(An exception to this rule is given by Lowell A. Glasgow et al.[99]
They found that murine— i.e., mouse—cytomegalovirus, which
is a relative of human cytomegalovirus, is far more effectively
combated when the drug acyclovir is administered orally than
when it is injected intraperitoneally. To cite a second example,
laetrile is active, for better or for worse, when taken orally, but is
without effect when administered by injection.[99a] Laetrile's
action is discussed in Chapter 5.) Thus, even if the same animal
(or human) model and the same dosage of the same nutrient or
drug were to be used in two experiments, but the method of
administration differed, the results might not be comparable. Be
wary of articles in popular magazines that may analyze a study
involving injection of a vitamin and then report that the vitamin
was "administered"—leaving the reader to erroneously assume
that the substance was taken by mouth.

The results of one study will sometimes be found to contradict
those of another. In such a case, it is likely that the experimental
protocols of those experiments differ in seemingly extraneous, but
actually important, factors that the respective scientists may, or may
not, have disclosed. John C. Bailar III[99b] discusses some of the

implications of well-done studies whose results are in conflict with each other.

It is not to be expected that a scientist will always be cognizant of the defects in the protocol of his study. What is important is that experimental details be fully disclosed so others may criticize the implications of that protocol. For example, a scientist doing studies of BHT-induced physiological damage in rats might not know that the cedarwood shavings used as bedding on the floor of the animal's cage could, through the sublimation of terpenes, and via an effect on the liver enzyme system, prevent BHT-caused lung damage. [100*] Thus, he might falsely conclude that BHT was innocuous from the standpoint of lung damage. Scientists making use of the possibly dangerous vehicles polysorbate 20, polysorbate 80, Tween 20 or Tween 80 for carrying vitamin E or other vitamins may improperly ascribe fetal malformations,[101] depressed immune response[102] and other outward effects[103] to the vitamin rather than to the vehicle. (More about the dangers of the polysorbates will be found in Chapter 2. Our concern at this point is only to point out that the toxic effects of the polysorbates could sometimes cause scientists to draw erroneous conclusions.) As long as a scientist fully discloses his protocol, others will have the opportunity to point out, in criticizing his research, that sesqui terpenoid compounds emanating from the cedar shavings might have protected the animals' lungs or that polysorbates may have caused toxic effects, contrary to the conclusions of the scientists conducting the respective studies.

As you read scientific literature, not only be on guard against possibly defective experimental protocols but beware of the experimenter's prejudices. A researcher may be so intent on proving

---

* Many physiological effects such as this occur through influences on the liver enzymes. Vesell et al.[100a] reported that not only aromatic hydrocarbons from cedarwood bedding, but also eucalyptol from aerosol sprays and chlorinated hydrocarbon insecticides can induce activity in the hepatic (liver) microsomal enzymes (HME). On the contrary, ammonia generated from feces and urine accumulated in unchanged pans under wire cages can inhibit HME activity. Rats in wire cages where the pans were changed infrequently had only one-third the aniline hydroxylase activity, a little more than one-half the ethylmorphine N-demethylase activity and two-thirds the cytochrome P-450 content of rats in wire cages where the pans were cleaned frequently. Vesell and his colleagues state that variations caused by the various above-noted factors in control animals can be so large as to obscure the effects being investigated in an experimental group.

his hypothesis that he could overlook alternate explanations of the phenomenon he is observing. Plaut quotes T. C. Chamberlin,[104] writing almost a century ago, who said, "The moment one has offered an original explanation for a phenomenon which seems satisfactory that moment affection springs into existence, and as the explanation grows into a definite theory his parental affections cluster about his offspring and it grows more and more dear to him." Be aware also that the scientist may have set his experimental parameters so as to make it impossible to discover a *reverse effect* (something we will be continuing to discuss throughout this book).

I hope this study of experimental protocol will help guide you. In order to sharpen your own talent for the criticism of experimental protocol, visit a medical library and consult *Citation Abstracts*. These volumes permit you to discover articles by various scientists that have referenced the study in which you are especially interested. The authors of these more recent articles may have comments on the validity of the study that concerns you.

This excursion into ways to more meaningfully read biomedical literature has two more subtle purposes. The first is to caution scientists about exposing their subjects (animals or humans) to stressful conditions that are not essential to the purpose of their studies. Secondly, and more important, I want to emphasize the fact that a person's health or illness is influenced (as are the health or illness of an animal in a laboratory cage) by many factors that may ordinarily escape our attention and the attention of our physicians.

"Nutritional questions have about them an air of reasonableness that often belies their intrinsic complexity. Nutrition is direct and personal for everyone, and nearly everyone, it seems, has an opinion on the subject. It is not surprising that controversy abounds, to say nothing of faddism, exploitation, and outright charlatanism."
— R. P. Heaney[1]

CHAPTER 1

How to Use the *Reverse Effect* and the *Pleasure Concept*

What is *health*? According to the constitution of the World Health Organization (WHO), health is a state of complete physical, mental and social well-being, not merely the absence of disease or infirmity.* Health is also a high-energy state accompanied by a feeling of being at peace with oneself and with others. To achieve and maintain good health we must have good nutrition. However, good health depends on far more than good nutrition.

For one thing, mental attitude can be extremely important. A study of four decades by George E Vaillant[4] showed the effect of mental health on physical health and longevity. A total of 204 men were selected as adolescents for continued study. Of the 59 men with the best mental health assessed from the age of 21 to 46 years, only two became chronically ill or died by the age of 53. Of the 48 men with the worst

---

* F. C. Redlich[2] disagrees with the WHO definition of health. He maintains that health is "nothing more than the absence of disease." Obviously, I am pro-WHO and anti-Redlich on this issue. Those who are philosophically inclined will want to read not only Redlich, but other articles in the same issue that carried Redlich's article and also one by Michael H. Kottow.[3] Kottow, in turn, cites references for additional study.

mental health assessed from the age of 21 to 48, 18 became chronically ill or died by the age of 53. Vaillant concludes that "good mental health retards midlife deterioration in physical health." The positive mental attitude toward one's illness and toward one's doctor is also of great therapeutic importance. S. Greer et al.[5] reported that, in a study of 69 breast cancer cases, the patient's psychological response was a significant factor in the course of the disease. They reported that, "Recurrence-free survival was significantly common among patients who had initially reacted to cancer by denial or who had a fighting spirit than among patients who had responded with stoic acceptance or feelings of helplessness and hopelessness." In a followup of the same patients about five years later, Keith W. Pettingale, Steven Greer et al.[5a] found that recurrence-free survival continued to be significantly more common among those who reacted with denial or "fighting spirit." Greer has quoted J. Paget[6] as saying (over 100 years ago), "The cases are so frequent in which deep anxiety, deferred hope and disappointment are quickly followed by the growth and increase of cancer, that we can hardly doubt that mental depression is a weighty addition to the other influences favoring the development of the cancerous constitution." Lawrence LeShan[7,8] has reviewed many studies showing the influence of mental state on the development of malignant disease. Additional studies involving the mind-cancer connection have subsequently been reviewed by Constance Holden.[9] Interestingly, Phillip Shaver et al.[10] reported that certainty of religious beliefs (either strong religiousness or confident nonreligiousness) was associated with better mental and physical health. It is apparent that good health and bad health are functions of the mental state.

The living of a healthy, vigorous life and the attainment of longevity will not simply occur. We must maintain a happy, friendly, confident attitude. We must like ourselves; we must give and receive love. We must eat good foods and when necessary, use additional nutrients in the form of supplemental vitamins and minerals and perhaps take them at certain times of the day or night. We must exercise regularly throughout our lives—and the exercise should, ideally, include regular, loving sexual activity. Furthermore, to live long, healthy lives our days must be filled with joy...not only with the joy of sex,* but also with the pleasure of eating and drinking, including perhaps an occasional cup of coffee, an alcoholic drink or a banana split. If one experiences great pleasure in eating or drinking a proscribed treat, I believe the benefit to the psyche will in many cases offset the negative nutritional aspects. In addition to the psychic value, there is the physiological effect of increased enzyme flow when eating or drinking is accompanied by feelings of pleasure. I call this idea the *pleasure concept.* Do not, however, eat or drink questionable foods at every meal and in between your meals.**

Hedonic capacity—the ability to experience pleasure—is a measure of health and can be important in influencing more usual ways of analyzing health status. Anhedonia—a severely limited capacity to experience pleasure—has been described as a characteristic of schizophrenia by many psychopathologists.[15-25a] A number of true-false type tests, including those of Loren J. Chapman et al.,[15] have been devised to measure anhedonia. More recently, Robert H. D. Dworkin and Kathleen Saczynski[21] have constructed scales of hedonic capacity from the Minnesota Multiphasic Personality Inventory and the California Psychological Inventory. Dworkin and Saczynski found significant positive correlations between hedonic capacity and responses to daily events such as feelings of elation/pleasure, playfulness, leisureliness and friendliness. They found significant negative correlations between hedonic capacity and feelings of anger, fear, sadness and annoyance. The *pleasure concept,* as I have

---

* Erik Agduhr[11] found that sexual activity increases resistance of both male and female rats, mice and rabbits to toxic substances. (Perhaps the rationale for this finding relates to stimulation of gonadotropin. Agduhr found that injecting gonadotropic hormone into unmated mice poisoned with arsenic also resulted in an antitoxic effect.) D. Drori and Y. Folman[12] reported significantly increased longevity in rats who had the opportunity to mate at least once a week. The results of a subsequent study by Drori and Folman[13] are shown in Figure 1.

** Nevertheless, let's not lose sight of the doctrine of "sufficient challenge."[14] Muscles, brains and sex organs are made stronger through challenges and perhaps other organs may also be benefitted. Might not small amounts of coffee or alcohol strengthen the liver? H. F. Smyth, Jr.[14] reported that rats inhaling small amounts of the poison carbon tetrachloride grew better and were more fertile than controls.

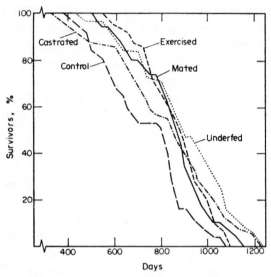

Figure 1. Survival of mated, exercised, underfed, castrated and untreated (intact) control male rats. Castration and underfeeding produced more *late* survivors, but exercise and mating prolonged life better while the males were young. Graph reproduced from D. Drori and Y. Folman, *Experimental Gerontology* (1976) 11: 25-32, with permission of the authors and of the publisher, Pergamon Press, Ltd.

presented it, suggests (to me) that the Dworkin and Saczynski scales of hedonic capacity will eventually be related to a great multitude of health-related problems other than depression and schizophrenia, and including longevity itself. Paul E. Meehl[22] has said: "I am convinced that 'high joy' people do exist; and I should be surprised if my readers, in contemplating their range of acquaintances, disagree with me. There are persons who seem able to take considerable pleasure from almost any circumstance not distinctly loaded with aversive components and for whom the most ordinary experiences appear to be a source of considerable gratification. I conjecture that these people are the lucky ones at the high end of the hedonic capacity continuum." In characterizing individual differences in hedonic capacity, Paul E.

Meehl[22] cites the Wild West maxim, "Some are born three drinks behind." Meehl goes on to say: "I think people with low hedonic capacity should pay greater attention to the 'hedonic bookkeeping' of their activities than would be necessary for people located midway or high on the hedonic capacity continuum. That is, it matters more to someone cursed with an inborn hedonic defect whether he is efficient and sagacious in selecting friends, jobs, cities, tasks, hobbies, and activities in general."

To many persons the search for good nutrition has become an unhealthful neurosis. To maximize health, I believe that the search for good nutrition must become not a neurosis, but a way of life. It must be a way of life in which one generally eats healthful food in pleasant surroundings with a congenial person or persons. But it will also be a way of life in which no guilt is attached to the occasional eating of a not-so-healthful fun-food just for the sheer pleasure of it.

Learn to intensify the pleasures of eating by savoring your food. Enjoy its color; note its texture. As you bring the food slowly to your mouth, excite your nostrils with its aroma. Good eating, like good sex, should have a loving period of foreplay. Chew every bite far more times than is usually considered to be necessary. Revel in the taste sensations. Make each act of eating an adventure in sensuality. Long-staying eating and long-staying sex have more benefits in common than is generally realized. There is an added advantage to super-enjoyment of food beyond this increase in psychic joy. Through getting all this additional pleasure from the food you eat, satisfaction is achieved sooner and overeating becomes merely a problem of yesterday.

It is widely believed, and I also hold this view, that fried foods are less healthful than the same foods prepared differently. However, a contrary view regarding the unhealthfulness of fried foods is suggested by some data from the *Hammond Report on Smoking in Relation to Mortality and Morbidity* that was presented by E. Cuyler Hammond, Sc.D. of the Medical Affairs Department of the American Cancer Society, New York, N.Y. to the American Medical Association in 1963.[26] This material was brought to my attention through reading an interesting book, *Wine of Life,* by Harold J.

Morowitz. The *Hammond Report* provides longevity data of a group of 442,094 men aged 40-89, over a period of 34.3 months. It indicates that both smoking and nonsmoking men who regularly eat fried foods seem to live longer than those who do not! Observe this interesting data at age-standardized death rates per 100,000 man-years during the 34.3 month period that was studied:

Age-Standardized Death Rates

Weekly Frequency of Eating Fried Food	Subject Never Smoked Regularly	Subject Smoked 20 Cigarettes or More Daily
No Fried Food	1,208	2,573
1-2 times	1,004	1,694
3-4 times	642	1,714
5-9 times	781	1,520
10-14 times	722	1,524
15 or more times	702	1,399

Reproduced from E. Cuyler Hammond, *Jrl. of the National Cancer Institute* (May, 1964) 32: 1161-1188.

I think it quite premature, however, to conclude that fried foods are more healthful.* This data from the *Hammond Report* provides, I believe, an example of the *pleasure concept* in operation. It is probable that persons who avoid fried foods may do so because they already have bad digestive systems and might tend to die earlier whether or not they ate such foods. Nevertheless, I believe the data also suggest, but of course do not prove, that those more casual about their eating habits—even if life-shortening foods are consumed—will generally live longer than those eating only healthful

---

* Stephen L. Taylor[27] of the University of Wisconsin, Madison, has found that foods deep-fried are far less mutagenic than foods cooked on a grill. The deep-fried foods, with their surfeit of fat, may add to heart problems, but it is the grilled foods that may pose a greater threat of cancer.

foods if the orientation of the latter group is such that pleasure is reduced.*

I suggest that those overly concerned about their eating habits have less fun in life. Those eating fried foods 15 or more times per week may, as a group, experience more joy in eating. Perhaps in other ways also they may find more pleasure in living *which is an approach to life that, I believe, promotes longevity.* Those who, on the other hand, can minimize their intake of fried foods without becoming overly concerned about such restrictions to the point that pleasure is reduced might, I think, live still longer. I believe it important that healthful foods be eaten more often and the consumption of unhealthful ones (including perhaps fried foods) be reduced *without one's pleasure being reduced.* In line with this reasoning, I suspect that an overconcern for eating presumably healthful foods such as yogurt, wheat germ and brewer's yeast on a rigidly regular basis could actually be life-shortening if it takes too much pleasure out of life. Eat healthful foods and avoid unhealthful ones, but only to the extent that such eating does not reduce the fun of living!

The beneficial effect of love in experiments with rabbits implies that love is also very important for human health and longevity. Robert M. Nerem et al.[28] reported that rabbits, on a 2% cholesterol diet, when petted, held, talked to and played with on a regular basis had improved health. Compared to control groups given the same diet, the experimental groups showed more than 60% reduction in percentage of aortic surface having sudanophilic lesions even though serum cholesterol, heart rate and blood pressure were comparable.**

---

* The beneficial effects of eating fried foods (like the benefits of modest drinking of alcohol) may also involve stimulation of the liver's microsomal enzymes, collectively called cytochrome P-450. (This will be discussed in Chapter 3.)

** B. S. Gow et al.[28a] and M. J. Legg et al.,[28b] using different strains of rabbits, were unable to replicate these results. (Nerem and his associates used the Sudan strain of New Zealand White rabbits while the Gow and Legg groups used Canadian and Australian strains of New Zealand White rabbits.) The "love-factor" in the development of atheroma in cholesterol-fed rabbits seems to depend on the strain of rabbits used. Perhaps the "love-factor" in human health may vary from person to person just as do the effects of vitamins and drugs. The concept of what I propose to call *amative individuality* may be just as valid as that of *biochemical individuality* which was popularized by Roger J. Williams and which we will be considering frequently in the pages ahead.

(When two scientists get conflicting results, could it sometimes be that only one is taking cognizance of the *pleasure concept*?)

When Michael Plaut et al.[28c] deprived rat litters of their mother at the age of 13 days, 90% of the adult-deprived pups died between 18 and 21 days of age. But, the scientists say, "most mortality was prevented by the presence of a nonlactating adult." They go on to comment, "Survival could be attributed largely to the opportunity for tactual contact between pups and the adult, even though a significant amount of mortality could be prevented even by housing maternally deprived pups with a female from whom they were separated by a double wire screen." Not the lack of mother's milk, but the absence of loving contact, or the absence, at least, of a nearby female, is what seems to have been the major cause of death. Elsewhere, Plaut [28d] has this to say in regard to undernutrition in young rodents:

> These studies provide support for the hypothesis that offspring physiology and behavior can be affected by adult-litter interactions which are not related to nutritional factors. This hypothesis is contrary to the tacit assumption, made in many studies of undernutrition, that the effects of maternal deprivation can be related only to nutritional factors. The hypothesis is substantiated by some studies of early weaning in which an additional group of pups is left with a mother whose nipples have been cauterized to prevent suckling. Where this was done, the effects of maternal deprivation were not seen in the offspring of the cauterized mothers.

Love and physical contact are "nutrients" essential to the well-being of rodents (and humans). The need for love can be readily seen in lower animals such as birds. It is interesting to speculate, since I believe the relevant studies have not yet been made, whether the need for love exists in worms, amoebae, bacteria and plants.

In a related study, W. B. Gross and P. B. Siegel[29] habituated chickens to human beings by talking to them, offering them food and gently handling them, a process called *socialization*. After seven weeks of socialization the birds were challenged by an exposure to *Escherichia coli*. Compared with ignored chickens, the socialized birds showed a 60% reduction in pericarditis and death. In another study, Gross and Siegel [30] found that when socialized chickens were stressed by fasting and then exposed to *Staphylococcus aureus* their resistance was good. However, when unsocialized chickens were given a similar treatment, their resistance was less.

Jay R. Kaplan et al. [31] performed a related experiment with monkeys. Thirty animals were assigned to six groups, each of which contained five members, and all were fed a moderately atherogenic diet. Group members were changed continually among three groups of five monkeys to create an unstable social condition, while the other three groups of five were allowed to remain in a stable social condition. Each of the 30 monkeys was classified as dominant or subordinate based on patterns of aggression or submission. Both dominant and subordinate animals in unstable social groups had significantly greater coronary artery atherosclerosis than those housed in stable social groups.

Social isolation among human groups can be similarly related to disease. John N. Edwards and David L. Klemmack[32] "found that the best predictors of life satisfaction are socioeconomic status, perceived health status and informal participation with nonkinsmen." Judith G. Rabkin and Elmer L. Struening[33] state that sheer size of a given group, called *ethnic density,* has been found to be inversely related to psychiatric hospitalization rates.

Michael G. Marmot and S. Leonard Syme[34] found that among men of Japanese ancestry, the gradient in occurrence of coronary heart disease (CHD) was lowest in Japan, intermediate in Hawaii and highest in California. They maintain that "this gradient appears not to be completely explained by differences in dietary intake, serum cholesterol, blood pressure and smoking." Marmot and Syme hypothesized that social and cultural values may account for the CHD differences between Japan and the United States. They classified 3,809 Japanese Americans according to the degree to which they maintained a traditional Japanese culture. The investigators found that in the most traditional group the prevalence of CHD was as low as that in Japan. The group most acculturated to Western living had a three- to five-fold excess in the prevalence of CHD. Marmot and Syme concluded that "this difference in CHD rate between most and least acculturated groups could not be accounted for by differences in the major coronary risk factors."

Analogous studies in the town of Roseto, Pennsylvania, which is ethnically homogenous, have also related inversely the prevalence of CHD with social support and close family ties. John G. Bruhn et al.,[35] who have analyzed nine of these studies, give us the lesson Roseto teaches:

> The major lesson from Roseto is that we all have a need for a safety net. We all have a need for ties that bind us to the social fabric. We need someone to talk to, to listen; we need social institutions, clubs, organizations, and informal groups to provide us with a sense of purpose for living; we need close personal ties with a loved one, with family members, and with others who care beyond listening; we need a philosophy or point of view of life to help us set personal goals and assess our personal ability to share, to give, and to take; and finally we need to select a physical and social environment in which to live that will provide a meaningful mixture of opportunities and security.

Pleasure can be affected by changes in life events, for better or for worse. Loss of a loved one, divorce or loss of a job can sometimes have negative effects on our health. Other life change events may (but will not necessarily) represent beneficial stresses, and some of these might be marriage, a new job or a vacation trip. Many studies[36-38] have found that clusters of events are associated with illness. Rafaella M. A. Osti et al.[39] reported that stressful life change events were associated with the occurrence of hypertension. Carol W. Buck and Allan P. Donner[39a] have also associated life change events with hypertension. Life change events have also been related to ischemic heart disease, myocardial infarction and stroke.[39b-e] Those making high scores on the Holmes-Rahe Social Readjustment Rating Scale[40] and on the UCLA Loneliness Scale have been reported by Janice K. Kiecolt-Glaser et al.[41] to have decreased immuno-competence as indicated by significant declines in natural killer cell activity and in total plasma IgA. In a subsequent study, Steven E. Locke et al.[42] found that life change stress and natural killer cell activity were not significantly correlated, but they reported that "good copers" had significantly higher natural killer cell activity than those who were not "good copers." R. W. Bartrop et al.,[42a] studying the effects of severe stress on the immune system of 26 bereaved spouses, found that the response to phytohemagglutinin and to concanavalin A was significantly depressed, but only after a delay of six weeks. S. J. Schleifer et al.[42b] reported, on the other hand, that lymphocyte function was immediately depressed after bereavement and persisted for two months or more.* Harold Levitan[42ba] recently reported that intense grief seemed to be a key psychological factor contributing to the onset of asthma. Life change events have also been associated with the development of *alopecia areata* (a kind of baldness),[43a] yeast infections,[43b] late onset manic-depressive disorder,[43c] rheumatoid arthritis,[43d] colds,[43e] gastric (but not colorectal) cancer,[43f] and appendicitis.[43g]

Kenneth P. Matheny and Penny Cupp[44] found that not only could negative life changes lead to illness but, in the case of females (but not of males), desirable events (if unanticipated) were also positively related to illness. Matheny and Cupp note that one of the factors that may contribute to the degree of life change stress is whether or not a given change was anticipated. Those who doubt their ability to cope may increase the negative effect of the anticipated change. On the

---

* Studies of widows and widowers show an increase as high as 40% in mortality rates compared to married men and women of the same age.[42c] Knud J. Helsing et al.[42d] reported that mortality rates among widowed males who remarried were much lower than among those who did not remarry. However, they found no significant difference among widowed females who did or did not remarry. Interestingly, Marian Osterweis et al. cite W. P. Cleveland and D. T. Gianturco[43] as reporting that age-specific mortality rates among widowed males who remarried were lower than the rates among married males.

other hand, self-confident persons may make plans to meet the anticipated change and thus reduce its stressing effect. Paul J. Rosch[45] points out that "pleasurable experiences may be powerful stressors, and winning a race or an election may evoke the same or greater secretion of epinephrine or hydrocortisone as losing; getting married is likely to be as stressful as becoming divorced." Therefore, "desirable" or "undesirable" events may have a stressing effect. We must not assume, however, that stress is always detrimental. Hans Selye[46] coined the word "eustress" to designate pleasurable stress as distinguished from "distress," meaning painful stress. It is not the type of stress, but the demands it places on us and our perceived capability of meeting those demands that are the determining factors. It is not so much the nature of stress nor whether the stress was or was not anticipated that detrimentally or beneficially affects our lives, but our perception of each of those stressors and our reactions to them. The support of family and friends and of our communities, and especially support of what Rickey S. Miller and Herbert M. Lefcourt[46a] call a "current intimacy" is vital to our well-being. Their offering consolation during times of bad stress and congratulations in times of beneficial stress add to life's pleasure and are health-fostering. When bad events occur, one with a "healthy personality" tends to express feelings such as anger,* hate, fear and sorrow if he has such feelings. The less healthy personality has similar feelings

---

* W. D. Gentry et al. [46b] found that those who showed a tendency to express the anger they felt had lower rates of hypertension than those who suppressed their anger. Steven Greer and Maggie Watson[46c] reported that independent groups of scientists [46d,e] have found expression of anger to be significantly less among breast cancer patients than among controls. Greer and Watson[46c] noted that similar findings have been reported by Watson et al.[46f] in patients with malignant melanoma. Anger, in my opinion, ideally should be directed against what was done rather than against the one who did it. One might say: "What you did has made me angry. Why did you do this?" Airing the grievance is, I believe, more healthful and gives the other person an opportunity to explain and perhaps to apologize. Aristotle is credited with saying, "Anyone can become angry—that is easy; but to be angry with the right person, and to the right degree, and at the right time, and for the right purpose, and in the right way—that is not within everybody's power and is not easy." Anger can modify many physiological parameters, including even the composition of the intestinal flora. L. V. Holdeman et al.[46g] have reported a variation of the composition of fecal bacteria in those under emotional stress. Specifically, during periods of anger or of fear stress there is a rapid increase in the level of *Bacteroides fragilis*, subspecies *thetaiotaomicron* in the ascending colon (perhaps arising, I presume, from action in the cecum). Subsequently, these bacteria are found throughout the colon.

but does not know in which direction to take those feelings. To have a good sense of personal worth, to feel in control of life rather than being controlled by life, to love more, to laugh more and to cry more when appropriate and to do "crazy" things sometimes—these are important for better health.[*]

We have seen many examples of the *pleasure concept* in action. Whether it is the rabbits being petted, chickens being socialized, monkeys living in stable groups or human beings living in socially close, loving communities, pleasure is a health-fostering factor. The nutritive power of love and pleasure is just as needed as are other forms of nutrition if we are to live healthfully and long. However, we have also seen that the golden mean of moderation, even in matters of pleasure, may be important in order to avoid psychological *reverse effects* just as it will be shown to be important in avoiding physical *reverse effects*.

In further relation to pleasure, the studies of Reubin Andres[48] and of A. R. Dyer et al. (the Chicago Peoples Gas Co. study)[49] indicate that a modest degree of overweight may be life-lengthening.[**] The favorable longevity effect of moderate drinking of alcohol has also been reported in several studies (as cited in Chapter 7). *The Boy Scout Handbook* gave (and perhaps it still gives) the advice, "Eat to live; don't live to eat." There is, of course, much to be said in favor of that statement. Although one should not live only to eat, I believe

---

[*] Many studies confirm the influence of mental attitude on health and disease while a few deny or minimize its importance. In keeping with the attitude expressed throughout this book, I want to encourage readers to investigate positions contrary to my own. If you are interested in studying denials of mental effects on physical health, ask your librarian to obtain an article by Marcia Angell[46h] and also some of the studies cited therein, especially those by Robert B. Case et al.[46i] and by Barrie R. Cassileth et al.[47] Recent reviews by Austen Clark[47a] and by Edward R. Friedlander[47b] are also interesting.

[**] R. J. Garrison et al.[50] have, however, criticized various weight-longevity studies because of failure to control for smoking. Leanness and smoking tend to be correlated. Thus, the factor of not smoking rather than the factor of overweight, itself, may have resulted in increased longevity. (Refer to a 1987 review by Manson et al.)[50a] Ulf Smith[50b] maintains that overweight persons with big abdomens are health-threatened more than those of similar weight and height whose fat is distributed around the hips and limbs. The abdominal fat pattern, according to Smith, carries a three- to five-fold increased risk of myocardial infarction or stroke. He says that a waist-to-hip ratio of over 1.0 in men or over .8 in women has a significant impact on prognosis.

that, unless one receives joy from eating, the lack of pleasure could be life-shortening. Pleasure, in moderation, is life-extending.[*]

Perhaps you have never felt the full intensity of the pleasure that you are capable of feeling. As an experiment, eat your food while concentrating on the sensations and compare the feelings you have with those experienced in ordinary eating. Try giving total concentration to smelling a flower, to looking at a painting—or to making love with such intensity that you are cognizant of nothing other than you and your lover's[**] oneness. I speculate that greater pleasure, whether attained in these or in other ways, will lead to less tension and increased health.

I speculate that some of us will be more healthy if our lives are filled with the joys of play, of travel and of being tuned in to the world of art, music, poetry, sports, politics and science. Others, however, will find that fixing their car, going to a bar or picking up women (or men) to be more pleasurable, and I speculate that for such persons these actions are health-fostering. I hold that laughter, conversation with friends, the wonder and delight shown by children, the smell of a rose or of dinner, sexual and nonsexual touching and hugging, red raspberries picked and immediately eaten, the face of a sleeping child, doing a good turn for someone with my role in the action being discovered only by accident, and a sense of unity with all of creation are joys that add to my pleasure. I believe that such experiences are, for me, health-fostering. Not just the experiences, but the memory of those experiences, add to the delight I take in living. I recall, as a 12-year-old, buying all the 5¢ Jamestown, U.S. postage stamps of 1907 I could find in dealer stocks at 25¢ each and the economic power I felt in selling them next year for $1.00 apiece. (I thus discovered for myself the profit-

---

[*] Bernard Fisher et al.,[51] in a randomized study involving 1,843 women, reported that segmental mastectomy (lumpectomy), *with or without radiation,* led to a higher disease-free survival rate than total mastectomy. (Segmental mastectomy with radiation was, however, greatly superior to the same operation without radiation.) Does this argue lumpectomy patients may feel happier than those who have had a breast removed? Is this yet another example of the longevity-increasing effect of pleasure?

[**] When I use the word *lover,* I do not exclude lovers married to each other. The term *lover,* as I use it, simply refers to one who loves.

making power behind what I call the *Law of Current Supply and Future Demand.*) I remember the intellectual "coming of age" that occurred through winning, against nationwide rivals, the University of Chicago's six-hour scholarship competition. I recall, as a young adult beginning to develop *dynamic synthesis,* how I used my entire "fortune" of $180 to trade stocks until my account was worth $5,000 (at which point I started a business). I remember the excitement, a few years later, in seeing a featured photo in the Decatur, Illinois, newspaper of one of my oil wells gushing uncontrolled over a field of soybeans. I recall the delight at the birth of my son Ron and of my daughter Pam. I remember my late wife and I designing our home and the subsequent pictures of our library that appeared in the *New York Times* and in other national media. I recall the flowers and wines of Madiera, the Great Pyramid of Cheops cutting a wedge of blackness in the star-filled Saharan sky, sunset behind the Parthenon and the visual treasury of a sunrise with Venus still shining through the already-blue sky. All of us have experienced our own versions of pleasure-yielding events, but do you and I extract all the pleasure possible from these life experiences?

To live most healthfully we must seek to live life more fully. Living life for some persons may mean a denial of most of what has been said above. For some, pouring a concrete sidewalk on a beautiful Sunday afternoon is just as pleasurable as a trip to an art institute may be for another. A photographer might derive more pleasure from working in his darkroom than he would from going on a picnic. The editing of this chapter is being done on a beautiful Sunday and is giving my editor and me a pleasurable sense of accomplishment. I speculate that for better health it is important to engage in pleasure-yielding activity enthusiastically—with maximization of its pleasurable possibilities.

Pleasure is a culturally-defined concept. It is based on society's concept of normative values. What is pleasurable today in socially unacceptable ways may, in the future, become socially acceptable. In the 1940s, oral sex was illegal in many states but now many enjoy it even though it is still on the books as being illegal. Nude sunbathing is similarly growing in acceptability. Our concept of pleasure today should not be unduly limited.

An important key to living healthfully and youthfully all one's life is to maximize the number of experiences that are apt to be worth experiencing. Perhaps to be most healthy we must continually experience the greatest joys of all. And what are the greatest joys of all? Each of us will have different ideas of such joys, but perhaps you'll agree with mine: the giving and receiving of love to and from a very special person and helping that person and all others with whom I come in contact to live happier, more meaningful lives. (If the health benefits of love could be provided by a pill, that pill would outsell all the vitamins and drugs on the shelves of drugstores and of health food suppliers.) In our giving and receiving happiness we should strive to achieve in ourselves, and foster in others, peace of mind.*

The *pleasure concept* of health deserves our attention not only in terms of *thought* but in terms of *action*. A most important prescription for health and longevity is to *determine what you like to do—what makes you very happy—and then find lots of opportunities to do it!*

Pleasure must, however, be subject to the dictates of the Greek principle of the *golden mean*. The *golden mean* recognizes that there is a position between "too little" and "too much" that is often superior to either extreme. Not only in the case of pleasure but in the case of various other phenomena, including the action of toxins and of nutrients, there is a *golden mean* that may be more healthful than either extreme. Science has a lot to learn about the quantities of nutrients or of toxins which are likely to lead to either health benefits or health threats. Like the love-hate duality to which human love affairs are subject, so there is a love-hate body reaction that may be exhibited by foods, vitamins, minerals, alcohol, coffee and other substances.

---

* An important step toward achieving and maintaining peace of mind is to keep a list of jobs to be done. Work on each item in the sequence of its time-order importance. Keep a the top of the list the never-finished project entitled: "Make love, not war."

The *Reverse Effect*

The *theory of the reverse effect* states that there is a good probability that any activity or any substance that is health-promoting or health-destructive in a given concentration may, on occasion, reverse its role and become respectively health-destructive or health-promoting at a different concentration. Furthermore, the same activity or the identical dosage of a substance may sometimes show an opposite effect in different persons or animals. What I term a *reverse effect* is not always a matter of going from enhancement to inhibition, but may simply be a trend reversal from increased enhancement to lesser enhancement or from increased inhibition to lesser inhibition. The action will be modulated* not only by the amounts of the chemical or other entity being considered but by the species involved, its health-disease state and its environment. In some cases (e.g., vitamins C and E) the *reverse effect* may involve a change in role from that of antioxidant to pro-oxidant. Perhaps the *theory of the reverse effect* will remind some of my readers of the statement of J. B. S. Haldane: "Nature is not only queerer than we suppose, but queerer than we *can* suppose."

The toxicologist, M. Alice Ottoboni[52] is referring to the phenomenon I call the *reverse effect* when she writes:

> Every toxicologist who has been engaged for any period of time in research into chronic toxic effects of chemicals has observed, more often than not, that animals in the group with the lowest exposure to the test chemical grew more rapidly, had better general appearance and coat quality, had fewer tumors, and lived longer than the control animals. I know from personal experience that novice

---

* Note my use of the word *modulated*. If the *reverse effect* concept proliferates, I suspect that, in the absence of dose-response data on a given substance relative to a given disease, scientists and physicians will increasingly employ the words *modulate* or *modulated* when an effect is apparent but it is not known if a given dosage works as a cause or as a cure or acts to exacerbate or to molify.

toxicologists usually consider such observations as aberrations in their data or the result of some flaw in their experimental design or conduct. They are usually loath to call attention to such findings, perhaps because to do so might bring their competence into question, or because they are unable to explain the reason for such findings. It is only with the confidence that comes with experience that the research toxicologist can comfortably acknowledge the occurrence of such results in his own experiments and broach the subject with his colleagues. The reaction from his fellow toxicologists is usually one of, "You, too?"

The phenomenon of beneficial effects from trace exposures to foreign chemicals, although often a subject of conversation among toxicologists, particularly with regard to why such effects occur, is rarely mentioned in the scientific literature. If the phenomenon does occur in a chronic toxicity experiment, the text of the paper reporting the results will seldom mention the fact. It is only by careful perusal of the data tables and figures presented in the body of the text that the phenomenon is revealed. Such subtleties are lost on people who read only the abstracts of scientific papers. Unfortunately, there are some scientists who may be counted among the abstract-only readers.

The doctrine of "sufficient challenge" of H. F. Smith, Jr.[14] was introduced in a subnote earlier in this chapter. This doctrine is based on the concept that an unused function atrophies. Ottoboni[53] quotes Smith as saying: "I think that most of the small non-specific responses which we measure in chronic toxicity studies at low dosages are readjustments or adaptations to sufficient challenge. I interpret them as manifestations of the well-being of our animals, healthy enough to maintain homeostasis. They are beneficial in that they exercise a function of the animal. Only when challenge becomes overwhelming does injury result." The doctrine of "sufficient challenge" obviously casts doubt on the attitude expressed by the Delaney Clause. The Delaney Clause is based on the idea that if a substance is carcinogenic in large dosages it may also be dangerous in small dosages and it should therefore not be permitted as a food additive. *The Federal Register*[54] perpetuates the line of reasoning behind the Delaney Clause by saying, "The exposure of experimental animals to toxic agents in high dosages is a necessary and valid method of discovering possible carcinogenic hazards in man." Those fostering the Delaney Clause are not concerned with the possibility that such "carcinogens" might, at certain dosages, constitute a "sufficient challenge" and offer protection against cancer. We will consider the Delaney Clause again later in this chapter.

In this book I will report on much research suggesting that large amounts of vitamins and minerals may at times be harmful. Conversely, I speculate that small quantities of toxins may beneficially stimulate the liver to be more efficient just as muscles become stronger when they are occasionally exercised.* The advice to eat a well-balanced diet may be good information not only in order to achieve a broad spectrum of needed nutrients but because it introduces the body to a well-balanced but minor intake of toxins, at least some of which in small amounts might actually be beneficial. Nutrition and pharmacology must become sciences, not merely of nutrients, drugs and toxins, but sciences of dose-response relationships.

Thus, I am suggesting that we do not always know which constituents are good and which are bad for the body. *That which is good may be bad; that which is bad may be good.* It depends on the circumstances and one of the circumstances is the quantity of the presumed nutrient or presumed poison that is involved. W. W. Duke,[55] three-quarters of a century ago, tested the effects on blood platelets of many different agents such as toxins, bacteria, a chemical

---

* The rationale for this proposed action may involve stimulation of the liver's microenzyme cytochrome P-450. This will be discussed in Chapter 3 (references 129b-d of Chapter 3).

poison and x-rays. He observed that agents causing rapid and large rises in the platelet count (diphtheria toxin and benzol) were the ones producing the most rapid and extreme falls in the count. It was an early recognition of the presence of a *reverse effect.*

Several decades later, Lawrence P. Garrod[56] gave examples of bacterial growth being stimulated when small dosages of chemotherapeutic agents were used. Among those examples he cited was a study of G. E. Foley and W. D. Winter[57] which showed that penicillin increased the mortality of chick embryos inoculated with *Candida albicans.* Garrod noted that "superinfections" sometimes occur clinically during penicillin treatment. On the other hand, T. D. Luckey[58] has reported that antibiotics such as sulfa drugs, succinylsulfathiazole, streptomycin and 3-nitro-4-hydroxyphenyl-arsonic acid can be used in very small quantities to support life and to promote growth in animals.*

About a quarter-century ago, N. V Medunitsyn[58e] found that various painful stimuli given rabbits had an influence on immunological reactivity. A weak stimulus increased phagocytic activity of the leucocytes and increased the antibody titer in the blood while strong painful stimuli showed a *reverse effect* and suppressed these processes. Alcohol in moderation can add to the joy of life and may possibly bring improved health and greater longevity. In excess, alcohol can produce liver cirrhosis and death. A high dose of not only alcohol, but also of sodium pentobarbital, acts as a behavioral depressant, while a low dose of either drug produces behavioral activation.[59] Small amounts of vitamin D are good—they help put

---

* However, antibiotics stimulate growth not only of the animals, but of the biota they are meant to oppose. In 1978, 48% of the antibiotics produced were designated for use in animal feeds.[58a] They are used not only for growth promotion but for better feed conversion, prophylaxis and the treatment of certain diseases.[58b] However, there is a danger in the practice. It appears that antimicrobial-resistant bacteria from animals can cause infection in humans and there have been a number of investigations of epidemics that may have been caused by these bacteria.[58c] Scott D. Holmberg et al.[58d] have identified 18 persons in four midwestern states that have been infected by *Salmonella newport,* a strain resistant to antibiotics. The onset of the illness was often triggered by the taking of amoxicillin or penicillin. They concluded that "antimicrobial-resistant bacteria of animal origin can cause serious human disease, especially in persons taking antimicrobials, and that the emergence and selection of such organisms are complications of subtherapeutic antimicrobial use in animals. We advocate more prudent use of antimicrobials in both people and animals."

calcium in the bones. Large amounts are bad—they pull calcium out of the bones and dump it in the soft tissues, including those of the kidney and of the joints.

Sometimes antivitamins can fulfill some of the functions of the vitamins they ordinarily oppose. Pantoyl taurine can, according to Robert E. Hodges et al.,[60] both cause a pantothenic acid deficiency or reverse that effect and mimic some of the properties of the vitamin. Hodges also reports that the antagonist *omega methyl pantothenic acid* may possibly act as a substitute for pantothenic acid in aiding production of antibodies, thus reversing its generally antagonistic nature. The two-faced nutritional and antinutritional properties of vitamins and their antagonists make the science of nutrition far more subtle than it was once thought to be.

Reverse effects are very common, albeit often unrecognized. Prolactin stimulates milk secretion in lactating women. Prolactin appears also to facilitate processes associated with sperm capacitation (the process, occurring in the vagina, by which sperm become capable of fertilizing an ovum).[61,62] A deficiency of prolactin may be associated with benign prostatic hypertrophy and nominal amounts seem to be required for prostatic health.[63] Rubin et al.[64] reported that prolactin seems to be capable of increasing plasma testosterone in adult men. Furthermore, according to S. P. Ghosh et al.,[65] rat experiments suggest that prolactin acts with testosterone to regulate acid phosphatase activity in the male accessory sex organs. * On the other hand, excessive prolactin, hyperprolactinemia, shows a *reverse effect* compared with normal amounts of prolactin and (like a deficiency of prolactin) is often associated with impotence, hypogonadism, decreased semen volume and reduced spermatic

---

* Interestingly, unless prolactin secretion increases in young (but not in older) men during sleep, their testosterone production is unlikely to follow its normal tendency to peak the following morning.[66] The herb yohimbine from bark of the evergreen tree yohimbe, often used as an aphrodisiac, may stimulate prolactin secretion.[67] (Scientists for many years have declared aphrodisiacs to be nonsense. Experiments at Stanford University by John T. Clark et al.[68] have shown that yohimbine has both immediate and more lasting effects in increasing the sexual appetite of male rats. Experiments are now underway at Stanford to test yohimbine's effect in men. Perhaps the results will confirm what African natives have maintained for centuries about the effects of using the bark of the yohimbe tree.)

density in men and lessened orgasmic capacity in women.[69-72] (Bromocriptine is often used to reduce prolactin levels and for bringing on a restoration of potency and of orgasmic capacity.) Thus, too little or too much prolactin may lead to dire sexual effects.

John Bancroft[72a] reported that L. Lidberg [72b,c] and, later, Lidberg and Sternthal[72d] found that oxytocin may enhance sexual responsiveness in men. Bancroft noted that two of the three studies showed the effect was greater at lower dosages and he refers to the results as "these surprising findings." It is another example of the *reverse effect.*

Pharmacists preparing anticancer drugs may become victims themselves according to a study at the M. D. Anderson Hospital, Houston, Texas.[73,74] The urine of nine pharmacists preparing such drugs became highly mutagenic showing that somehow they absorbed substances that mutate cells, leading possibly to cancer and thus exemplifying the *reverse effect.* A number of other studies[75-78] have reported that urine of nurses and other hospital personnel handling cytotoxic drugs showed positive mutagenicity. Smoking may potentiate the hazard.[77] Recently, Marja Sorsa et al. [77a] published additional evidence of the hazards of occupational exposure to anticancer drugs. Many others have commented on the problem.[79-82*] Then too, a *reverse effect* of the cytotoxic drugs may be shown in the cancer patients themselves after they have been "cured." Robert Hoover and Joseph F. Fraumeni, Jr.[82c] observe that various alkylating agents (including not only cyclophosphamide but also melphalan and chlorambucil) used in treating malignant neoplasms can all *cause* cancer (perhaps, in part, because they break chromosomes). Lancet[81] comments, "In patients who have been cured of malignant disease, clinicians gloomily accept that further neoplasia may arise as a late effect of treatment." Would this occur as

---

* The antineoplastic drugs (cyclophosphamide, diethylstilbestrol, fluorouracil, methotrexate and vincristine) show teratogenic and mutagenic *in vivo* effects in animals. Selevan et al., [82a] in a case-control study involving 17 hospitals in Finland, found that pregnant nurses exposed to antineoplastic drugs had a statistically significant increase in fetal loss. Nurses who lost their fetuses were twice as likely to have been exposed to antineoplastic drugs during the first trimester as those who gave birth. In a related article, Bingham[82b] has observed that, "Institutions such as hospitals and university laboratories have not been in the forefront of occupational-disease prevention."

often if the therapies took full cognizance of dose-related *reverse effects?*

Small amounts of an allergen may stimulate Immunoglobulin E (IgE) antibody production, whereas larger amounts of that allergen may suppress such production.[83] E. R. Stiehm et al.[84] reported that the alpha, beta and gamma families of interferons, which are produced when mammalian cells are stimulated in the inflammatory process, can augment the immune function or can show a *reverse effect* by suppressing immunity. Interferon has the ability to inhibit growth of some malignant cells. On the other hand, a study by Gene P. Siegal et al.[84a] showed that at least three types of interferon can *increase* the ability of Ewing sarcoma cells to invade healthy tissue, which also exemplifies the *theory of the reverse effect.* And so it is in the case of many other drugs, vitamins and minerals.

Foods can also display *reverse effects.* Frederick Hoelzel and Esther DaCosta,[85] in reporting that a protein-deficient diet caused ulcers to form in the stomach and duodenum of mice, observed that an excess of protein also tended to produce gastric lesions. Then too, water sustains life and also displays the *reverse effect* of causing death by drowning.*

Reverse effects are also very common where radiation is concerned. T. D. Luckey[86] relates that small amounts of radiation seem to increase the reproduction rates of protozoa. Fecundity of higher animals may also increase with increased radiation, hens may lay more eggs and sterility rates may be reduced. Luckey cites studies showing that irradiated mammals have increased cerebral blood flow, brain development, audio and visual acuity and learning ability. Large amounts of radiation show a *reverse effect* and cause a decrease in various life functions; still larger amounts result, of course, in death. Many studies, also cited by Luckey, indicate that background radiation can reduce deaths attributed to cancer, while

---

* Even excessive amounts of drinking water may be dangerous to epileptic patients. White[85a] observes that hydration has long been known to induce seizures. He calls attention to a diet plan which advocates drinking of eight to twelve 8-ounce glasses of water per day and cautions that epileptic patients should be aware of the possible dangers.

larger amounts show a *reverse effect* and, as is well known, can cause cancer.*

The *Encyclopaedia Britannica*[87] states that, "A sample of nearly 100,000 survivors of Hiroshima and Nagasaki yielded the anomalous result that groups exposed to doses between 11 and 120 rads actually had a lower death rate in the ensuing 15 years than those receiving a lesser dose." (It is anomalous only in the sense that there is little appreciation for how common the *reverse effect* really is.) A more recent analysis by G. W. Beebe et al.[88] found similar but somewhat different results. Beebe et al. showed a death rate during the 25-year span of 1950-1974 of 23.3% for persons who received no radiation, then rising death rates up to 25.5% at a dose level of 99 rads. At a level of 100-199 rads a *reverse effect* set in and death rates declined to 23.8%, declined further to 22.6% at 200-299 rads, and further yet to 21.6% at 300-399 rads. Then a second *reverse effect* occurred and at dosages of about 400 rads the death rate was highest at 28.4% (as expected). It is interesting to note that the death rates for those exposed between 200 and 399 rads were lower than controls that received no radiation.

Exposure of plants and animals to x-rays and other ionizing radiation shows many beneficial effects. L. P. Breslavets et al. [89] reported that irradiating dry seeds of the radish and the carrot at 2,000 to 4,000 rads before sowing increased radish production by 11% and that of carrots by 26%. The carotene content of the carrots increased by 57%. L. D. Carlson et al.[90] found that rats exposed to low total-body irradiation of .1 rad/hour for 8 hours daily from 4 months to 16 months of age had increased life spans. They speculated that mild injury may be beneficial by stimulating renovation processes. Radiation may even be useful in human therapies. Carolyn Ferree[90a] has reported that the occurrence of gynecomastia (abnormal growth of breasts) secondary to estrogen

---

* Radiation from the sun and from the rest of the cosmos has been bombarding life on earth for the two billion years life has existed. Recently, the intensity of some types of radiation that reach earth has diminished due to the presence of particulates from industrial pollution. Other types of radiation have probably increased due to reduced protection provided by the ozone layer. Could it be that optimal radiation for living things are those levels existing before man fouled the atmosphere?

therapy for prostatic cancer can be largely prevented by irradiating each breast with 900 to 1,000 rads before estrogen therapy.

Roy E. Albert et al.[91] reported many interesting dose-response relationships of beta-ray-induced skin tumors in rats. Figure 2 shows

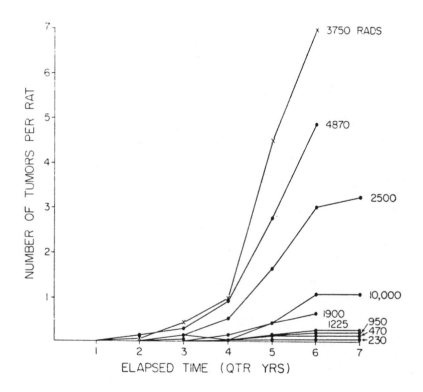

Figure 2. Cumulative incidence of adnexal tumors in rats versus elapsed time after irradiation. Note that the number of tumors increased up to an irradiation level of 3,750 rads and then showed a *reverse effect* by declining at 4,870 rads and declining further at 10,000 rads. Graph reproduced from Roy E. Albert et al., *Radiation Research* (1961) 15: 410-430, with permission of the publisher, Academic Press. (This graph exemplifies the fact that sometimes data can be presented in such a way as to mask the *reverse effect*. See Figure 3.)

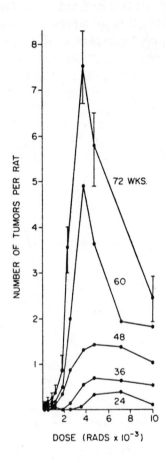

Figure 3. Skin tumors of all types (adnexal, epidermoid carcinoma, etc.) per rat versus skin irradiation dose at the indicated post-irradiation times. Bar lines indicate standard error. Data presented in this form more clearly show the *reverse effect* than do the data presented in Figure 2. Graph reproduced from Roy E. Albert et al., *Radiation Research* (1961) 15: 410-430, with permission of the publisher, Academic Press.

the cumulative incidence of adnexal tumors per rat at three-month intervals for various dosages of radiation. Note that the smaller dosages from 230 to 1,900 rads produced very few tumors. The most tumors developed at a level of 3,750 rads. Then a *reverse effect* set in with fewer tumors being produced at 4,870 rads and fewer still at 10,000 rads. Figure 3 shows the total number of skin tumors of all types as a function of radiation dosage. It is a method of presentation that more clearly shows the *reverse effect*.

Wheeler P. Davey[92] similarly observed that beetles exposed at two different moderate dosages of x-radiation lived longer than controls not exposed at all, those exposed at low dosages and those exposed at high dosages. Many such experiments are cited by T. D. Luckey.[93]

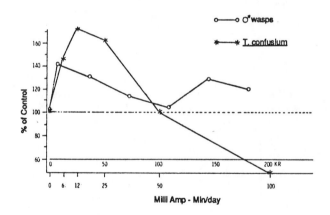

Figure 4. Increased longevity in invertebrates exposed to x-rays followed by a *reverse effect* and lowered longevity. The data of Davey exhibit the response of *T. confusium* to mA/min/day of radiation. The abscissa for the data of Sullivan and Grosch with male wasps is given in kR as one acute exposure. Graph reproduced from T. D. Luckey, *Hormesis with Ionizing Radiation* (Boca Raton, Florida: CRC Press, 1980), with permission of the publisher.

T. D. Luckey's book[93] contains some very interesting graphs, three of which are shown here. Figure 4, using data from Davey[92] and from R. L. Sullivan and D. S. Grosch,[94] shows that the life span of the insect *Tribolium confusum* increased to a maximum at an x-ray exposure of about 12 milli amp/min/day and then a *reverse effect* set in, reached par with controls at 50 milli amp/min/day, and then continued to show longevity decreases. The same figure illustrates the response of male wasps to radiation expressed   as   kR   and   given

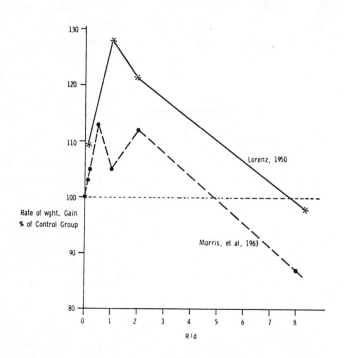

Figure 5. Increased growth rates in irradiated mice were comparable in experiments of different laboratories. In both cases, after an initial surge, a *reverse effect* set in, followed by decreased growth rates. Graph reproduced from T. D. Luckey, *Hormesis with Ionizing Radiation* (Boca Raton, Florida: CRC Press, 1980), with permission of the publisher.

as one acute exposure. Here, the life span increased at an exposure of about 10 kR, then showed a *reverse effect* by declining almost to a par with controls at about 55 kR. At this level a *biphasic reverse effect* set in with longevity increasing again as the radiation dosage was raised.

Figure 5, again from Luckey,[93] illustrates different experiments by E. Lorenz et al.[95] and by J. J. Morris et al.[96] on growth rates in mice irradiated with x-rays. These experiments indicate maximum growth as the radiation increased from .1 to .5 or 1 R/day. At about .5 or 1 R/day (depending on the study) *reverse effects* occurred and rate of weight gain declined, reaching par of the control group at 5 to 7.5 R/day and then continued to worsen.

Figure 6, the final illustration from Luckey,[93] shows yields of grain and of strawberries in terms of x-ray dosages based on data from studies by L. P. Breslavets and A. S. Afanasyeva,[97] by R. K. Schulz[98] and by I. Fendrik.[99] Growth increased as x-ray dosage rose and reached maxima (in some cases doubling the yield of the controls) between 10^2 and 10^3 R/day. Then *reverse effects* took place and, between a radiation level of 10^3 and 10^4, the yield declined to par of the controls and then continued to decline as dosage increased.

Concern has been expressed about the dangers of electromagnetic waves emanating from high tension wires and questionable tales have been told about the Russians using such waves to "zap" our embassy in Moscow. One of the effects of electromagnetic waves on cells is to affect the glucose content. Crediting the work of Budho, A. S. Pressman[100] of the Department of Biophysics, Moscow University, Moscow, U.S.S.R., has illustrated the phenomenon with two graphs (Figures 7 and 8). Note (in Figure 7) as the frequency of the waves increases glucose content of cells declines, but at 30 k Hz a *reverse effect* sets in and thereafter the glucose content rises. A similar effect is shown as the field strength varies. Glucose content declines as field strength increases up to about 15V/cm, then shows a *reverse effect* and rises as the field strength continues to increase (Figure 8). From these examples it should be apparent that *reverse effects* are common when life forms interact with radiation.

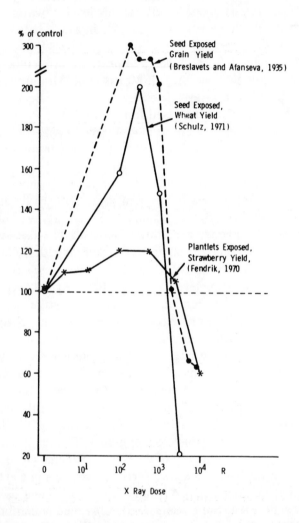

Figure 6. Changes in yield as seeds and plants are irradiated. In each case, a *reverse effect* is apparent. Graph reproduced from T. D. Luckey, *Hormesis with Ionizing Radiation* (Boca Raton, Florida: CRC Press, 1980), with permission of the publisher.

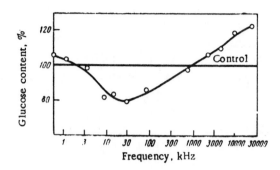

Figure 7. Change in glucose content of isolated rat liver due to low- and high-frequency EmFs. Note the *reverse effect* at about 30 kHz. Graph reproduced from A. S. Pressman, *Electromagnetic Fields and Life* (New York: Plenum Press, 1970) pp. 156-157, with permission of the publisher.

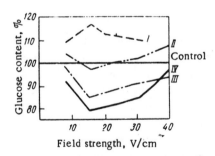

Figure 8. Change in glucose content of isolated rat liver in relation to EmF strength. I) 9.5 MHz; II) 730 kHz; III) 85 kHz; IV) 29 kHz. Note the *reverse effect* at about 15 V/cm. Graph reproduced from A. S. Pressman, *Electromagnetic Fields and Life* (New York: Plenum Press, 1970) pp. 156-157, with permission of the publisher.

Paracelsus, back in the 1500s, is credited with the statement, "Dosis sola facit venenum—Only the dose makes the poison." Then in the 19th century, a principle in pharmacology was developed that came to be known as the *Arndt Law* or the *Arndt-Schultz Law.* This law states: *weak stimuli excite physiologic activity, moderately strong ones favor it, strong ones retard it, very strong ones arrest it.* T. D. Luckey has been a key factor in the development of the related sciences of *hormology* and *hormoligosis.* Luckey has defined *hormology* as the study of excitation and includes in it not only the effect of *hormones* but the effect of other chemicals, radiation, heat, cold and other agents on cells. Hormoligosis is the part of hormology which includes the entire phenomenon of the stimulatory effect of a small amount of an agent on living organisms. *Hormesis* is the subdivision of hormoligosis which deals with the stimulatory amount of toxins, and the compounds involved are called *hormetics.** In connection with hormology, Luckey has modified the Ardnt-Schultz Law to read: *subharmful doses of any harmful agent may stimulate organisms in suboptimum condition.* Luckey[102] predicts, by the way, that "over half of all toxic compounds would be hormetics if appropriately low doses were administered."

The *theory of the reverse effect* differs from the Arndt-Schultz Law and from hormology in that it relates to organisms that are not necessarily in a suboptimum condition and it recognizes that the effect of a "high dosage" is often not simply a matter of retardation or arrest, but one of producing an opposite effect. Weak or moderate sexual activity may increase the functional ability of a man's prostate gland. Too much sex, on the other hand, might not merely arrest the prostate's ability to perform (as the Arndt-Schultz Law might suggest), but could induce a pathological condition that might be attended by symptoms of pain and bleeding. Vitamins C and E can not only act as antioxidants (as is well known) but, as we noted earlier, can show a *reverse effect* by acting as pro-oxidants. (See Chapters 2 and 6.) Many examples of the *reverse effect* can be found throughout this book.

---

* The word *hormesis* was neologized by C. M. Southam and J. Ehrlich who reported [101] that an extract of tree bark stimulated bacteria at low levels but was bacteriostatic at high levels. Luckey has expanded their definition.

As I said, a chemical or other entity (e.g., exercise or pleasure-yielding activity), which at a given dosage causes a certain physiological reaction, will often cause a *reverse effect* at either a much greater or a much smaller dosage. Mild exercise (a "nutrient") may lead to a stronger heart, stronger arms, etc. Too much exercise, however, may at times bring on a heart attack and "tennis elbow" and, as we will see in Chapter 10, may even be life-shortening. Modest amounts of sunshine can foster health; large amounts can promote sunburn, leathery skin and melanoma. Other "nutrients" and "toxins" that exemplify *reverse effects,* in addition to exercise, drugs, herbs, vitamins, minerals, foods and pleasure-yielding activity, will probably occur to the reader.

With this line of reasoning, I am, of course, casting doubt on the multitude of experiments in which huge doses of a given substance are fed animals in order to produce, say, cancer and then those experiments are used to predict the possibility that the substance may cause cancer in man. I am not, right now, concerned with the dubious assumption that a chemical in the diet of man will act as that chemical does in the diet of a mouse. I am concerned, instead, with something I believe to be far more important. The procedure of estimating low-dose human response based on experiments involving high-dose animal response could be an improper extrapolation of dose-response relationships. The famous Delaney Clause,* as we noted earlier, is based on the presumed validity of this extrapolation that I am questioning. Extrapolation of any data outside the observable range can be an error-fraught exercise. M.

---

* Since the Delaney Clause was enacted in 1958, it has been interpreted to mean that no substance known to cause cancer in animals may be added to food. (It might be naturally present, but may not be added.)[103] Saccharin was subsequently given a legal exemption. In June, 1985, Dr. Frank Young, FDA commissioner, stated that his reading of the law permits use of the legal concept known as *de minimus,* meaning "the law does not concern itself with trifles."[103a] Young maintains that a *de minimus* risk does not mean the substance must be banned. Two articles by Marjorie Sun,[103b,c] one by Kessler[103d] and one by Flamm[103e] discuss some of the problems occasioned by the Delaney Clause.

Alice Ottoboni[104] tells about a "megamouse" study of the National Center for Toxicological Research (NCTR)[105] involving more than 24,000 mice and the carcinogen 2-acetylaminofluorene (AAF). A committee of the Society of Toxicology [106] reviewed the NCTR report.[105] Ottoboni, in citing from this review, said:

> The Society's review points out that the statistical model used for extrapolating effects from very low doses "provides statistically significant evidence that low doses of a carcinogen are beneficial...."
>
> "If the time-dependent low-dose extrapolation models are correct," the Society states, "then we must conclude that low doses of AAF protected the animals from bladder tumors." However, the Society also asserts, "...not only is the simple model used by NCTR statisticians inappropriate to the data, but most of the models that have been proposed in the statistical literature are also inappropriate." They urge a "profound rethinking of the entire problem of chemical carcinogenesis and low-dose extrapolation."

The *theory of the reverse effect* suggests just the opposite of the standard line of reasoning. Small doses of a huge-dose cancer-causer might protect against cancer! Tomorrow's statements of physiological interactions with drugs and nutrients are likely to be elucidated in dose-response tables rather than in simple sentences.

Then too, the fact that many drugs have side effects corresponding with the same condition for which they are curative provides many examples of the *reverse effect*. This fact also serves as a warning that drugs must be carefully studied for dose-responses and possible *reverse effects* that can be exacerbative rather than curative. If you study several drugs in the *Physicians' Desk Reference* [107] you will probably discover that, for at least a few of them, the list of side effects contains a symptom for which the drug is sometimes curative. The diazepam, Valium® is one such drug.* Among the indications for its use is included "management of anxiety disorders or for the short-term relief of the symptoms of anxiety." Among its adverse reactions are included "hyperexcited states" and "anxiety."[107b] The barbiturate, Nembutal® Sodium is used as a "sedative hypnotic." Among its side effects are "agitation," "nightmares," "nervousness" and "anxiety."[107c] Quinidine sulphate (Quinora®) is used for "paroxysmal atrial tachycardia" and "paroxysmal atrial fibrillation" and "paroxysmal ventricular tachycardia when not associated with complete heartblock." Among its adverse effects are "ventricular tachycardia and fibrillation" and "paradoxical tachycardia."[107d] The rauwolfia product, Harmonyl® is employed for its "antihypertensive effects" and it also displays "sedative and tranquilizing properties." Among its adverse effects are "nervousness," "paradoxical anxiety" and "nightmares."[107e] To cite a final example, Asellacrin®, a growth hormone (somatropin or somatotrophin) which is used in treating short children in the attempt to increase their height, may sometimes be subject to a *reverse effect*. The *Physicians' Desk Reference* relates that "bone age must be monitored annually during Asellacrin® administration, especially in patients who are pubertal and/or receiving concomitant thyroid replacement therapy. Under these circumstances, epiphyseal maturation may progress rapidly to closure."[107f] In other words, sometimes there is a *reverse effect* and, instead of the child growing taller, his epipheses close and he completely stops growing.

In each of these drugs the normal action shows a *reverse effect* at some concentrations in some persons. A *reverse effect* of the drug diphenylhydantoin (Dilantin®), alias phenytoin, involving vitamin D is shown in Chapter 4 and, in connection with hypertension (in the potassium section of Chapter 7), we will note the *reverse effect* shown by hydrochlorothiazide. At a given dosage a

---

* The patent on Valium® has recently run out, so there are likely to be many more diazepam drugs to offer it competition. Horrobin[107a] speculates that diazepams and possibly the benzodiazepines, including chlordiazepoxide hydrochloride (Librium®), may promote tumor growth. (Tumor promoters do not usually cause cancer when used alone but can enhance the effect of a cancer initiator.) Is it possible that diazepams and/or benzodiazepines at some dosage might show a *reverse effect* and act to cure cancer?

drug may *cause* in one person the same condition which the same dosage *cures* in another. A different dosage will often show a *reverse effect* and be curative to the first but detrimental to the second. The side effects of many of the drugs listed in the *Physicians' Desk Reference* give testimony to the reality of the *reverse effect.* Medicine, like nutrition, must study dose-response relationships and, by administering individually determined dosages in therapeutic applications, strive to eliminate iatrogenic *reverse effects.** (The research-minded reader will discover other *reverse effects* in the *Physicians' Desk Reference* and may also desire to search for additional examples in *AMA Drug Evaluations* [107fa] or in *Drug Facts and Comparisons.* [107fb] Some libraries also have on-line data base information regarding recently discovered drug-associated problems. If your local library does not have *Drug Facts and Comparisons* and its monthly supplements, your pharmacist may let you look at his.)

Let me caution against quickly concluding that small doses of a given substance may often be beneficial with large doses of that substance being dangerous. As we will see in Chapter 6, small amounts of vitamin C detrimentally encourage lipid peroxidation, larger amounts beneficially act as an antioxidant and still larger amounts may once again act detrimentally as a pro-oxidant. Studies show that estrogen can promote carcinogenesis. On the other hand, Joseph Meites et al.[107g] have shown that a large dose of estrogen (20 mg. of estradiol benzoate) effectively inhibited growth of DMBA-induced mammary tumors in rats. Meites also cites the work of C. Huggins[107h] and of R. I. Dorfman[107i] that also showed large doses of estrogen resulted in tumor regression in rats. In addition, Meites cites a study of J. Hayward[107j] in which large doses of estrogen (or of androgen) induced remission of human breast cancer in more than 20% of treated patients. In further regard to estrogen, Hoover and Fraumeni[82c] cite three studies that suggest oral contraceptives may

---

* Studying the *Physicians' Desk Reference (PDR)* at intervals of a decade or more, I get the impression that drugs reported by the *PDR* as having a "paradoxical effect" are associated with a tendency to be retired. However, a phenomenon is paradoxical only until the paradox is resolved. Would it be beneficial to keep using some of these retired drugs but more clearly define dose-response relationships?

offer some protection against ovarian cancer. Perhaps in the case of the ovary, estrogen may show a *reverse effect* at the dosage of the Pill and provide protection. Obviously, more (in the case of estrogen) may sometimes induce a beneficial *reverse effect.*

Large amounts of dihomo-gamma-linolenic acid (DGLA), a substance which is present in human milk and which is metabolized in the body (especially if evening primrose oil is consumed), can inhibit the growth of malignant cells *in vitro.* However, Robinson and Botha (as discussed in Chapter 3) found that a small amount (50 μg. per ml) of DGLA, on the other hand, can produce a *reverse effect* (my language) and promote cancer. Here again, a large amount of a substance may work for our benefit while a small dosage may be dangerous. (Since evening primrose oil is widely sold, it is important that any possible *reverse effect* be precisely delineated. In Chapter 3 we will consider evening primrose oil—its benefits and possible dangers—in greater detail. The *reverse effect,* as we will see throughout this book, can be very subtle indeed.)

Physicians must learn that the answer to ineffectiveness of a therapy is not necessarily to increase the dose. A decreased dose, instead, might produce the desired result. Similarly, scientists must learn to construct experimental protocols that make it possible to discover *reverse effects.* Often experiments are done with dosage increments that make it impossible to discover what, if any, phenomena might exist at intermediate levels.

Could the *theory of the reverse effect* have implications as a research tool, e.g., in the search for anticancer agents? Podophyllotoxin from the herb *American mandrake (mayapple)* is reported to cause cancer. It is reported to also actively inhibit carcinoma and sarcoma in animals. Perhaps it might prove rewarding to look for cancer-treating substances among factors known to be mitogenic, mutagenic or carcinogenic. Such a search might be a valuable application of the *theory of the reverse effect.* Mary E. Caldwell and Willis R. Brewer[108] recently published a list of 50 plant extracts from 42 species that have been shown to significantly enhance tumor growth. A total of 300 extracts were found to exhibit prominent enhancement of tumor growth. The work was well done in terms of its objectives and tests were performed at various toxic and nontoxic levels. However, I think the entire group of 300 extracts should be studied for *reverse effects* and possible antitumor action at some yet-to-be-discovered dosages.*

The *Reverse Effect* as a New Therapeutic Paradigm

Thomas S. Kuhn has thrown interesting new light on the ways in which various sciences evolve. Paramount to Kuhn's viewpoint is the role in scientific research played by "paradigms" which he defines as "universally recognized scientific achievements that for a time provide model problems and solutions to a community of practitioners."[108c]

Kuhn develops the thesis that "normal science," as he calls it, presupposes one or more paradigms which are accepted by practicing scientists as being beyond questioning. Thus, research tends to be looked upon as an act of puzzle-solving that occurs within the bounds set by a paradigm rather than as a free-wheeling exploration of the unknown. Kuhn, in his thought-provoking book *The Structure of Scientific Revolutions,* says:

> ...normal science repeatedly goes astray. And when it does—when, that is, the profession can no longer evade anomalies that subvert the existing tradition of scientific practice—then begin the extraordinary investigations that lead the profession at last to a new set of commitments, a new basis for the practice of science. The extraordinary episodes in which that

---

* D. R. Stoltz et al.[108a] found that 22 fruits and vegetables had mutagenic activity. Grapes, onions, peaches, raisins, raspberries and strawberries showed the most potent mutagenicity. Could components (perhaps flavonoids) from these six be concentrated to act as anticancer agents, as the *reverse effect* suggests? Many flavonols found in foods are mutagenic and references for this finding are found in Chapter 6. I have not seen studies indicating that 3,4'-dimethoxy-3'5,7-trihydroxyflavone and centaureidin are mutagenic and/or carcinogenic. However, S. Morris Kupchan and E. Bauerschmidt[108b] found that these flavonols from the plant *Baccharis sarothroides* showed significant inhibitory activity against cells derived from human carcinoma of the nasopharynx carried in cell culture.

shift of professional commitments occurs are the ones known in this essay as scientific revolutions. They are the tradition-shattering complements to the tradition-bound activity of normal science.[108d]

Kuhn, in further development of his view of "normal science," goes on to say:

Few people who are not actually practitioners of a mature science realize how much mop-up work of this sort a paradigm leaves to be done or quite how fascinating such work can prove in the execution. And these points need to be understood. Mopping-up operations are what engage most scientists throughout their careers. They constitute what I am here calling normal science. Closely examined, whether historically or in the contemporary laboratory, that enterprise seems an attempt to force nature into the preformed and relatively inflexible box that the paradigm supplies. No part of the aim of normal science is to call forth new sorts of phenomena; indeed those that will not fit the box are often not seen at all. Nor do scientists normally aim to invent new theories, and they are often intolerant of those invented by others. Instead, normal-scientific research is directed to the articulation of those phenomena and theories that the paradigm already supplies.[108e]

Thus, dramatic new breakthroughs can occur only through the process of overthrowing well-established doctrines. The doctrine that extrapolation can predict effects in nutrition and in medicine must be viewed as being obsolete. A *reverse effect* might be present and produce a reaction quite the opposite from what data extrapolation would suggest—perhaps even a cure from a known disease-causer. I

propose that the *theory of the reverse effect* as a tool for developing
new therapies is a revolutionary paradigm.

Orthodox nutrition and orthodox medicine have played too many
tricks on those relying on the efficacy of extrapolation for predicting
effects out of the range of available data. Nature is always a
formidable opponent. John Pfeiffer, in his excellent book regarding
radio astronomy, has this to say about the battle between nature and
science:

> Science is an intricate guessing game with nature as
> the adversary. The rules and regulations of the game
> are known somewhat loosely as the scientific
> method; the moves and strategies are our
> experiments and theories. Nature is continually
> fooling us, outguessing us, surprising us by doing
> the things we least expect of her. But every time we
> are fooled, we learn another one of her tricks. She is
> infinitely resourceful, of course, and we might as
> well face it.
>
> But we are fairly resourceful, too. When nature
> outguesses us, when we find our theories inadequate
> to account for the facts, we must be ready to shift
> and vary our attack as cleverly as a prizefighter
> exploring the strengths and weaknesses of his
> opponent.[108f]

So, it is time to conclude that the possibility of *reverse effects* should
be employed in devising nutritional and medicinal approaches for the
creation of new therapies.

Much "mop-up" work, as Kuhn would call it, will be needed to
determine *reverse effect* levels of different therapeutic agents for
various diseases. If, for example, mutagenic agents may work not
only to *cause* cancer but, at different dosages work to *cure* cancer,
what are the critical dosages for each such agent? Specifically, what

might be the cancer-fighting dose of each of the bioflavonoids that, at a different dosage, show mutagenicity? Are "miracle" cures a possibility? St. Augustine (354-430A.D.) said, "Miracles are not contrary to nature but only contrary to what we know about nature." It is time to employ the *reverse effect* as a new therapeutic paradigm. The existence of a vast body of anomalies following from the established paradigm of extrapolation demands a revolutionary approach and this new paradigm providing for possible *reverse effects*.

The *theory of the reverse effect* gives added support to the idea of eating a well-balanced diet: not too much of this, not too little of that. Then too, I think of the *pleasure concept* as being a sub-principle of the *theory of the reverse effect*. Occasional ingestion of coffee and sweet rolls or occasional sex may be psychologically nutritional. Too much coffee, sweet rolls or sex may be toxic. It is an application of the ancient Greek principle of the golden mean: *moderation in all things*. Now that we have speculated about the *reverse effect,* it may be useful to rephrase the *pleasure concept* as follows: *A generally beneficial substance consumed without pleasure or when one is in an angry state or is in unpleasant surroundings may be detrimental to the body. A generally detrimental substance consumed with joy may be beneficial to the body.*

Whenever dosages of nutrients can be shown to display *reverse effects* on body functions, the science of nutrition needs to be rewritten in terms of dose-response relationships. To the extent that relevant *reverse effects* exist, never again will the science of nutrition—whether a "nutrient" be defined as a food or a toxin, a mineral, a vitamin, sunshine or other radiation, sex or other exercise or pleasure, etc.—be the same.

Is there a rationale that might explain the *reverse effect?* A. J. Clark[109] postulated the existence of two types of receptor sites, one producing a positive effect and the second acting in opposition to the first. E. J. Ariens et al.[110] and J. M. von Rossum et al.,[111] as well as W. D. M. Paton[112] developed this idea further. It is theorized that at low concentrations a given substance combines mainly with the activating receptor. At higher concentrations the action of the activating receptor reaches a plateau or continues to increase to only a minor degree. On the other hand, the blocking receptor becomes increasingly more active and eventually the effect is to overwhelm the action of the activating receptor. The peak of the bell-shaped dose-response curve is reached, then passed and we have a *reverse effect*. Some substances may occupy only activating receptors or only blocking receptors. They would, of course, have linear dose-response curves and would not exhibit the *reverse effect*. Such substances that occupy only activating receptors may be far more rare than is now believed to be the case. It might, for example, be argued that aflatoxin, which is toxic in just a few parts per billion, depending on the species, and continues to be toxic at higher concentrations, might be such a substance. However, can we rule out the possibility that, in minute concentrations of say a few parts per trillion or per quadrillion,* aflatoxin might show one or more *reverse effects* and might even be therapeutic? I think much is to be gained from hypothesizing that most substances taken into the body or produced by the body will, at some dosage or dosages, show one or more *reverse effects*.

Scientists often find that for which they look, and I think they should be looking for *reverse effects*.** Even in cases where chemicals are not obviously involved (e.g., exercise and pleasure-activation) they may in actuality be involved. For example, exercise involves adenosine triphosphate (ATP), adenosine diphosphate (ADP), creatine, creatine phosphate, glucose, insulin, lactic acid, glycogen, etc.

---

* Scientists may soon be able to detect a single atom or a single molecule by laser-based analytic methods.[112a]

** In general, scientists find only that for which they are searching, serendipitous discoveries being rather rare. In attempting to set an appropriate dosage for a clinical trial of retinyl acetate for use in treating histopathologic lesions of the cervix, Seymour L. Romney et al.[113] wrote: "The 3 mg. dose was eliminated as part of the empiric effort to establish the maximally tolerated dosage." It seems obvious they gave no thought to the possibility that the 3 mg. dose could be more effective than the 9 mg. dosage they finally decided to use. (That is, no thought was given the possibility that a *reversal* could exist somewhere between a dose of zero and one of 9 mg.) The scientific literature contains innumerable other examples indicating that the possibility of a *reverse effect* was simply not considered.

Pleasure (or pain which, depending on its intensity, may sometimes be pleasurable) may involve endorphins and enkaphilins. Thus, the binding-site theory may have general application in explaining the *reverse effect*. In the case of cancer applications, mutagens that will modify the DNA of normal cells and sometimes produce cancer, may act reversely to combat cancer by modifying the cancer cell's DNA. Through this mechanism the function of a cancer cell may be inhibited leading, in turn, to its demise. The fact that normal cells may be destroyed concomitantly is regrettable but not crucial since the body can replace them through its normal reparative processes. Other explanations of specific *reverse effects* are suggested throughout the book.

Current nutritional and medical practice frequently ignores not only the possible occurrence of *reverse effects* but also generally ignores the importance of the time of day, time of month or time of year that a nutrient, a drug or other treatment is administered. The developing science of chronobiology is concerned with the fact that the toxicity and/or effectiveness of drugs (and also perhaps of nutrients and other treatment modalities) can vary greatly depending on the time they are administered. The possibly increased effectiveness of vitamins or of drugs administered on a nonuniform time basis is illustrated by studies of Erhard Haus et al.,[114] F. Halberg et al.,[115] L. E. Scheving et al.[116] and Karel M. H. Philippens.[117] Some of these scientists [114] observed that mice inoculated with L1210 leukemia survived for a statistically significant longer span when four courses of arabinosyl cytosine were administered at 4-day intervals—not in courses consisting of 8 equal doses at 3-hour intervals, but in sinusoidally varying 24-hour courses, the largest amount being given at the previously mapped circadian and circannual times of peak resistance to the drug. Other studies have also demonstrated the increased therapeutic effectiveness of sinusoidal dosage schedules. Such research suggests that drugs presumably having an unacceptable toxicity-therapeutic ratio may be useable and of considerable value when administered in accordance with chronotherapeutic principles.

Healthful Thoughts and Other Supplements

This book deals not only with the prevention of *disease,* but also with far more. Beyond just prevention of disease, this book relates to the building of *health.* Health is a state of well-being which is far superior to the mere absence of disease and relates to joy, happiness and the enhancement of life; and remember this: joy, happiness and the enhancement of life cannot only be the *result* of superior health but a *cause* of superior health. Most persons now believe in the reality of psychosomatic disease. Why not also believe in the reality of psychogenic health? You can think yourself into better health. Do it!

Often the comment is heard that if one eats good food, then supplementation is unnecessary. There are several reasons why this doctrine is apt to be false. Try as we can, it is unlikely that all our foods will be grown on rich soil, and thus at least some of these foods are less likely to contain the healthful array of minerals our ancestors enjoyed. Even if our foods were all grown on rich soil, many would still be irrigated with polluted waters and exposed to air pollution. Furthermore, we are breathing that polluted air and we are subjected not only to toxic chemicals in our foods but to those in cosmetics, cleaning compounds, and so on. Then too, our society subjects us to many mental stresses which may, if we let them influence us negatively, deplete vitamin and mineral stores as the body attempts to compensate for those stresses.

G. Brubacher et al.[118] make the point that borderline vitamin deficiency exists in many population groups and in single persons even in industrialized countries. Their studies demonstrated that the avoidance of pork and whole wheat bread can lead to a borderline vitamin B_1 deficiency. Similarly, their studies have shown that avoidance of other items can lead to other vitamin deficiencies. Most persons who have fully operational food-assimilational and enzyme systems can probably get their vitamin and mineral needs from their diet if their objective is an *average* state of health. Those less efficient in food assimilation and in enzyme production or those with unusual diets (such as those who avoid pork and whole wheat bread) or those desiring superlative health may require supplements.* Moreover, R. L. Gross and P. M. Newberne,[119] in citing C. M. Leevy et al.[119a] who studied a selected municipal hospital population, say:

> These studies of isolated vitamin deficiencies lead to the inescapable conclusion that a single nutrient deficiency can result in profound impairment of specific immunologic processes—a concept that has not yet received widespread attention or general acceptance. This inattention may be having important clinical results, since the immunologic defects resulting from even marginal deficiencies may significantly alter disease course and/or therapeutic response. The incidence of hypovitaminosis discovered in a randomly selected U. S. hospital population in the 1960's dramatically illustrates that this is not an exclusive problem of underdeveloped countries. In this study, only 12% of the 120 patients had normal serum levels of all vitamins tested; 88% had at least one deficiency, and 59% had two or more biochemical deficiencies. There appeared to be no consistent trend with regard to sex, age, or racial group. Only 39% of the deficient patients had any history of dietary deficiency, the other 61% consuming what was considered a normal U. S. diet. Clinical signs of deficiency were present in only 38%; the remainder had deficiencies falling into the subclinical or marginal categories.

The elderly may be especially prone to vitamin deficiencies. D. J. Smithard and M. J. S. Langman[120] found subclinical vitamin C

---

* On the other hand, it may be possible that food itself could sometimes supply a dangerous *excess* of vitamins. Certainly, Eskimos consuming bear liver have been known to get dangerous excesses of vitamin A. Kummerow maintains, as we will see in Chapter 4, that foods may contain unhealthful excesses of vitamin D.

deficiency in nearly half of geriatric patients they studied. Vitamin C, through its effect on the P-450 enzyme system (which will be discussed in later chapters), is a factor in drug metabolism. Thus, low levels of vitamin C in many of the elderly may account for their generally slowed rates of drug metabolism. One must, however, use caution in concluding that low levels of vitamins and/or minerals in the elderly are necessarily unhealthful. Remember, in any study of the elderly, the subjects have been selected on the basis of longevity. Some of their characteristics obviously account for that longevity. Which ones?

Vitamins can sometimes correct or partially correct for inborn errors of metabolism. These errors of metabolism involve genetically determined absences of, or reductions of, enzyme activity and almost any biological transformation could be affected. K. Bartlett,[120a] in a very thorough treatment (with over 300 references), takes each vitamin in turn and discusses vitamin-responsive inborn errors of metabolism. S. Harvey Mudd[121] has also discussed various phases of vitamin-responsive genetic disease. In this regard, Charles Scriver[122] tells of some of the ways in which a vitamin dependency caused by gene-dependent nutritional disorders could be operating. First, an abnormal gene product might affect the body's ability to convert a vitamin into its biologically active coenzyme. Secondly, the cells could be impaired in their ability to take up a vitamin to convert it to its coenzyme. Thirdly, the apoenzyme might be altered so as to impair its ability to bind to the coenzyme. The mutant allele (one of a pair, or of a series, of variants of a gene having the same locus on homologous chromosomes) might not completely eliminate activity at a particular step in the biosynthetic pathway. It might still allow some coenzyme to be formed if the precursor vitamin were present in sufficient concentration. Do you or I perhaps have an undiscovered mutant allele affecting a physiological phenomenon that might be helped by extra amounts of one or more of the vitamins?*

An excellent overview relating to gene-dependent disorders was written by S. Harvey Mudd[123] and is entitled "Vitamin-Responsive

---

* In Chapter 5 we will examine the possibility that megadoses of the B vitamins might in some cases play a detrimental role in the formation of enzymes.

Genetic Abnormalities." Mudd says: "...rather than there being a single 'ideal' human with a 'normal' requirement for a vitamin, about which actual persons cluster as imperfect approximations, there may well exist an array of individuals in any population with genetically determined differences in their vitamin requirements spread over a wide range. If this is so, determination of nutritional standards for vitamins takes on an increased complexity to which nutritionists may wish to give a good deal of thought in the years to come."

Every individual, whether or not he has genetic "abnormalities," is unique in his or her nutritional requirements. Drs. E. Cheraskin and W. M. Ringsdorf, Jr.[124] relate that between two healthy young men of the same racial stock, one may require 4.5 times as much calcium as the other and 6.5 times as much of a particular amino acid as the other. For some nutrients the range of minimums is probably much greater. Vitamins A and C are two such examples. One individual might require ten times as much of one or both of these vitamins as another person. However, Drs. Cheraskin and Ringsdorf (and, for that matter, Dr. Roger J. Williams in his many writings over a period of many years) should have observed that "biological individuality" applies inversely as well. The level at which a given vitamin or other nutrient may become toxic could be ten times *lower* in you than it may be in me.

This book should not be construed as giving medical advice. No vitamin, mineral, herb, food, drug or doctor ever "cures" any condition. The body cures itself when it receives the necessary raw materials and/or the necessary treatment. Furthermore, it should be emphasized that one's state of health and potential for great longevity depend on a multitude of factors, among which are: someone to love and be loved by; a good self-concept, an active sense of responsibility for one's own health; a positive attitude; a recognition of the fact that there are always options; a happy, tranquil mind with good ability to cope with stress, including efficient use of anger to get jobs done rather than to cause ulcers and heart trouble; a firm resolve to worry only about things one can conceivably control; a willingness to see problems as being opportunities; crying more, smiling and laughing more and in other ways expressing rather than holding back the emotions; giving attention to the needs of others; adequate exercise; sufficient rest; clean air;* pure water; wholesome food and all the necessary vitamins and minerals. The facts conveyed in this book must speak for themselves and are to be used or ignored in accordance with the independent judgment of each individual reader.

Often we hear criticism of the RDA (Recommended Dietary Allowances) which are set, at five-year intervals, by the Food and Nutrition Board of the National Academy of Sciences. In criticizing the RDA we should keep in mind that the ninth edition of the academy's book states:

> RDA are recommendations for the average daily amounts of nutrients that *population groups* should consume over a period of time. RDA should not be confused with requirements for a specific individual. Differences in the nutrient requirements of individuals are ordinarily unknown. Therefore, RDA (except for energy) are estimated to exceed the requirements of most individuals and thereby to ensure that the needs of nearly all in the population are met. Intakes below the recommended allowance for a nutrient are not necessarily inadequate, but the risk of having an inadequate intake increases to the extent that intake is less than the level recommended as safe.
>
> RDA are recommendations established for *healthy* populations. Special needs for nutrients arising from such problems as premature birth, inherited metabolic disorders, infections, chronic diseases, and the use of medications require special dietary and therapeutic measures. These conditions are not covered by the RDA.[125]

---

* Clean air obviously includes avoidance of smoking and smoke-filled rooms. However, smoking can improve some conditions. Through an anti-estrogenic effect, it reduces the incidence of endometrial cancer in postmenopausal women. [124a-c] Smoking may also help protect against ulcerative colitis[124d] and Parkinson's disease. [124e]

Henry Kamin was the chairman of the Committee on Dietary Allowances of the Food and Nutrition Board in charge of preparing the tenth edition of the book, *Recommended Dietary Allowances,* publishing of which was recently aborted.* Kamin has stressed that the RDA of vitamins and minerals are in accordance with their requirements as nutrients and without consideration of possibly desirable pharmacological effects. He says:

> ...it is not inconceivable that some nutrients, even *within* the limits of a normal varied diet may, by some chemical accident, have some beneficial effect unrelated to its normal biological function. There has been considerable activity recently which suggests that some compounds chemically related to vitamin A—but not necessarily having biological vitamin A activity—may act as anticarcinogens. Future RDA committees and perhaps—even at our limited stage of knowledge—our own, must consider and debate whether there may be benefits, unrelated to normal biological activity, which could accrue by changing the recommended level of a nutrient in a diet while still remaining within the normal dietary. But if it falls outside of those limits, then I think that it's a problem for pharmacologists rather than for RDA Committees. And, as we consider these possible

---

* On October 7, 1985, the National Academy of Sciences killed this report that was five years in the making because of an impasse between the authors and its reviewers in the academy. The report proposed to lower the RDA for vitamins A and C. Eliot Marshall,[126] writing in *Science,* says that Kamin thinks Frank Press, president of the Academy, "caved in to pressure from activists worried about the RDA's." Marshall reports that critics denounced the draft as a threat to welfare programs. A new committee will be formed to again consider possible revisions in the RDA. The failure by the National Academy of Sciences to publish the 1985 RDA Committee's report continues to be discussed. See, e.g., letters by Kamin,[127] by Robert E. Olson[128] and by Frank Press[129] as well as articles by Schneider et al.,[130] by Herbert,[131] and a group of articles by many authors in *Nutrition Today.*[132] A recent statement of the Food and Nutrition Board [133] regarding the scientific issues related to establishing the RDA is especially valuable. (This article also lists names and addresses of the 1986 members of the board.)

secondary benefits, we should also be careful to give
close attention to possible long-term risks.[134]

In the chapters ahead we will be examining the RDA for various
vitamins and minerals and pointing out cases where the RDA might
be set too low (e.g., calcium).* It will become clear that I personally
have no problem with one's decision to use amounts of nutrients that
may, in some cases, exceed the RDA. I also have no problem with a
decision to sometimes take in *less* than recommended amounts of
certain nutrients—examples being fatty acids and protein.** I think
"optimal nutrition" can refer to amounts that may be more or may be
less than the RDA. Pharmacological dosages of vitamins and
minerals in excess of RDA levels may have benefits and may pose
dangers. We will be exploring those benefits and those dangers in
the chapters to come. Now, together, we will examine overwhelming
proof in the case of vitamin after vitamin, mineral after mineral, that
each, depending upon dosage, can either help or harm the body.

The BIG Book

If this Sampler stimulates your curiosity, consider ordering
copies of the BIG book for yourself as well as for scientific and
health-minded family members and friends, using the form on
page 103. Also consider donating copies to libraries, using the
form on page 101.

---

* The possible need in many persons (especially women) for supplemental calcium is
being actively debated. The dangers as well as the benefits of greater calcium
consumption are discussed in Chapter 7.

** RDA values may vary from country to country.   The U.S. RDA for ascorbic acid is
60 mg., compared with 50 mg. in Holland and only 30 mg. in the United Kingdom.[135]

Introduction—153 References

1. Peter Mc Cullagh, *Medical Jrl. of Australia.* (1985) 142: 328–329.
1a. Adolph Grünbaum, *Psychological Medicine* (1986) 16: 19–38.
1b. Michael L. Burr, *Human Nutrition: Applied Nutrition* (1984) 38A: 329–334.
2. Philip W. Lavori et al., *New England Jrl. of Medicine* (1983) 309, no. 21: 1291–1299 at 1291–1292.
3. Thomas A. Louis, *Annual Review of Public Health* (1983) 4: 25–46.
4. John C. Bailar III et al., *New England Jrl. of Medicine* (1984) 311, no. 3: 156–162.
5. Lincoln E. Moses, *New England Jrl. of Medicine* (1985) 312, no. 14: 890–897.
6. S. A. Barnett and J. Burn, *Nature* (1967) 213: 150–152. Cited by S. Michael Plaut, *Pediatric Clinics of North America* (1975) 22, no. 3: 619–631, at 626.
7. Robert Ader, *Psychosomatic Medicine* (1980) 42, no. 3: 307–321, at 312.
7a. *Neural Modulation of Immunity*, ed. Roger Guillemin, Melvin Cohn and Theodore Melnechuk (New York: Raven Press, 1985).
7b. *Psychoneuroimmunology*, ed. Robert Ader (New York: Academic Press, 1981).
7c. *Mind and Immunity: Behavioral Immunology*, ed. S. E. Locke and M. Hornig-Rohan (New York: Praeger, 1983).
7d. *Mind and Immunity: Behavioral Immunology (1976–1982) An Annotated Bibliography* by Steven Locke and Mady Hornig-Rohan (New York: Institute for the Advancement of Health, 1983).
7e. *Stress, Immunity and Aging*, ed. Edwin Cooper (New York: Marcel Dekker, Inc., 1984).
7f. *Psychoneuroimmunology*, ed. Steven E. Locke et al. (Hawthorne, N.Y.: Aldine Pub., 1984).
7g. J. Edwin Blalock, *Jrl. of Immunology* (1984) 132, no. 3: 1067–1070.
7h. Jean L. Marx, *Science* (1985) 227: 1190-1192.
8. Marvin Stein et al., *Science* (1976) 119: 435–440.
9. Nicholas Pavlidis and Michael Chirigos, *Psychosomatic Medicine* (1980) 42, no. 1: 47-54.
10. Jay R. Kaplan et al., *Science* (1983) 220: 733–735.
11. R. H. Gisler et al., *Cellular Immunology* (1971) 2: 634–645.
12. Stanford B. Friedman et al., *Psychosomatic Medicine* (1965) 27: 361–368. Cited by Robert Ader, *Psychosomatic Medicine* (1980) 42, no. 3: 307–321, at 314.
12a. Steven Greer, *British Jrl. of Psychiatry* (1983) 143: 535–543.
13. Benjamin H. Newberry et al., *Psychosomatic Medicine* (1972) 34, no. 4: 295-303.
13a. Lawrence S. Sklar and Hymie Anisman, *Science* (1979) 205: 513–515.
13b. Madelon A. Visintainer et al., *Science* (1982) 216: 437–439.
14. Benjamin H. Newberry et al., *Psychosomatic Medicine* (1976) 38, no. 3: 155–162.
15. Andrew A. Monjan and Michael I. Collector, *Science* (1977) 196: 307–308.
16. Malcolm P. Rogers et al., *Jrl. of Rheumatology* (1983) 10, no. 4: 651–654.
17. Marcus M. Jensen and A. F. Rasmussen, *Jrl. of Immunology* (1963) 90: 17-20.
17a. I. S. Chohan et al., *Thrombosis and Haemostasis* (1984) 51, no. 1: 22–23.
18. Ernest A. Peterson, *Jrl. of Animal Science* (1980) 30: 422–439.
18a. P. Rachootin and J. Olsen, *Jrl. of Occupational Medicine* (1983) 25: 394–402. Cited by Donna Day Baird, *JAMA* (1985) 253: 18: 2643-2644.
19. Vernon Riley et al. in *Psychoneuroimmunology*, ed. Robert Ader (New York: Academic Press, 1981) pp. 45-46.
19a. Marcus M. Jensen and A. F. Rasmussen, *Jrl. of Immunology* (1963) 90: 21–23.
19b. A. R. Turnbull et al., *British Jrl. of Surgery* (1975) 62: 657.
19c. George F. Solomon et al., *Proc. of the Society for Experimental Biology and Medicine* (1967) 126: 74-79.
20. J. F. Spalding et al., *Laboratory Animal Care* (1969) 19, no. 2: 209–213.

21. John Nash Ott in *Environmental Variables in Animal Experimentation,* ed. Hulda Magalhaes (Lewisburg: Bucknell University Press, 1974) pp. 39–57.
22. James T. Marsh et al., *Science* (1963) 140: 1414–1415.
23. Susan R. Burchfield et al., *Physiology & Behavior* (1978) 21: 537–540.
24. Benjamin H. Newberry and Lee Sengbusch, *Cancer Detection and Prevention* (1979) 2, no. 2: 225–233.
25. Malcolm P. Rogers, *Arthritis & Rheumatism* (1980) 23, no. 12: 1337–1342.
26. H. M. Weiss et al., *Jrl. of Comparative and Physiological Psychology* (1976) 90: 257–259. Cited by Lawrence S. Sklar and Hymie Anisman, *Psychological Bulletin* (1981) 89, no. 3: 369–406, at 358.
27. F. H. Bronson and B. E. Eleftheriou, *Jrl. of Gerontology* (1965) 20: 239. Cited by James P. Henry et al., *Psychosomatic Medicine* (1971) 33, no. 3: 227–237.
28. B. L. Welch and A. S. Welch, *Proceedings of the National Academy of Sciences* (1969) 64: 100. Cited by James P. Henry et al., *Psychosomatic Medicine* (1971) 33, no. 3: 227–237.
29. George F. Solomon et al., *Psychotherapy and Psychosomatics* (1974) 23: 209–217.
30. Vernon Riley, *Science* (1975) 189: 465–467.
31. P. Ebbesen and R. Rask-Nielsen, *Jrl. of the National Cancer Institute* (1967) 39: 917–932.
32. David A. D'Atri et al., *Psychosomatic Medicine* (1981) 43, no. 2: 95-105.
33. Stanford B. Friedman and Lowell A. Glasgow, in *Health and the Social Environment,* ed. Paul M. Insel and Rudolf H. Moos (Lexington, Mass: D. C. Heath and Co., 1974) pp. 169–191, at 175. Originally appeared in *Pediatric Clinics of North America* (May, 1966) 13, no. 2: 315–335.
34. Ethel Tobach and Hubert Bloch, *American Jrl. of Physiology* (1956) 187: 399–402.
35. Howard B. Andervont, *Jrl. of the National Cancer Institute* (1944) 4: 579–581.
36. O. Muhlbock, *Acta Int. Union Against Cancer* (1951) 7: 351. Cited by Richard C. LaBarba, *Psychosomatic Medicine* (1970) 32, no. 3: 259–276.
37. J. L. Barnett et al., *General and Comparative Endocrinology* (1981) 44: 219–225.
38. Vernon Riley, *Science* (1984) 212: 1100–1109.
38a. Joseph T. King et al., *Proc. of the Society for Experimental Biology and Medicine* (1955) 88: 661–663.
39. Doreen Berman and Barbara E. Rodin, *Pain* (1982) 13: 307–311.
40. G. S. Wiberg and H. C. Grice, *Science* (1963) 142: 507.
41. James P. Henry et al., *Psychosomatic Medicine* (1975) 37, no. 3: 277-283.
42. James Rollin Slonaker, *American Jrl. of Physiology* (1935) 112: 176–181.
43. E. P. Durrant, *American Jrl. of Physiology* (1935) 113: 37.
44. David R. Lamb et al., *Laboratory Animal Care* (1966) 16, no. 3: 296–299.
45. H. M. Bruce, *British Medical Bulletin* (1970) 26: 10–13.
46. S. Michael Plaut et al., *Psychosomatic Medicine* (1969) 31: 536–552.
47. V. Riley and D. Spackman, *Proc. Amer. Assn. Cancer Res.* (1979) 18: 173. Cited by M. Chevedoff et al., *Food and Cosmetic Toxicology* (1980) 18: 517–522, at 521.
48. June Marchant, *British Jrl. of Cancer* (1967) 21: 576–585, at 584.
49. Patricia F. Hadaway et al., *Psychopharmacology* (1979) 66: 87–91.
50. George F. Solomon et al., *Nature* (1968) 220: 821–822.
51. G. Newton et al., *Jrl. of Nervous and Mental Disease* (1962) 134: 522. Cited by ref. 50.
52. S. Levine and C. Cohen, *Proceedings of the Society for Experimental Biology and Medicine* (1959) 102: 53. Cited by ref. 50.
53. Stanford B. Friedman et al., *Psychosomatic Medicine* (1967) 29, no. 4: 323–328.
54. Robert M. Nerem and Murina J. Levesque, *Science* (June 27, 1980) 208: 1475–1476.
54a. Robert Ader and Stanford B. Friedman, *Jrl. of Comparative and Physiological Psychology* (1965) 59, no. 3: 361–364.
55. Robert Ader, *Psychosomatic Medicine* (1970) 32, no. 6: 569–580.

56. Stephen H. Vessey, *Proc. of the Society for Experimental Biology and Medicine* (1964) 115: 252–255.
57. David E. Davis and John J. Christian, *Proc. of the Society for Experimental Biology and Medicine* (1957) 94: 728–731.
58. Paul Brain, *Life Sciences* (1975) 16: 187–220.
59. P. D. McMaster and R. E. Franzl, *Metabolism* (1961) 10: 990. Cited by Stanford B. Friedman and Lowell A. Glasgow in *Health and the Social Environment,* op. cit. (ref. 33) p. 175.
60. E. D. Kilbourne et al., *Nature* (1961) 190: 650. Cited by Stanford B. Friedman and Lowell A. Glasgow in *Health and the Social Environment,* op. cit. (ref. 33) p. 175.
61. I. E. Bush, *Pharmacological Reviews* (1962) 14: 317. Cited by Stanford B. Friedman and Lowell A. Glasgow in *Health and the Social Environment,* op. cit. (ref. 33) p. 176.
61a. W. Cassell et al., *Proc. of the Society for Experimental Biology and Medicine* (1967) 125 supp.: 676–679.
61b. B. Jencks, unpub. doctoral dissertation, University of Utah (1962). Cited in ref. 61a.
62. F. H. Bronson and B. E. Eleftheriou, *General and Comparative Endocrinology* (1964) 4: 9 as cited by John W. Mason, *Psychosomatic Medicine* (1968) 30, no. 5. (Part III): 576–607, at 579.
63. J. W. Mason, J. V. Brady and M. Sidman, *Endocrinology* (1957) 60: 741, cited by John W. Mason, *Psychosomatic Medicine* (1968) 30, no. 5: (Part III) 576–607 at 579.
64. Robert Ader and Nicholas Cohen, *Psychosomatic Medicine* (1975) 37, no. 4: 333–340.
64a. Robert Ader et al., *Trends in Pharmacological Sciences* (1983) 4, no. 2: 78–80.
65. Michael Russell et al., *Science* (1984) 225: 733–734.
66. S. Michael Plaut, *Pediatric Clinics of North America* (1975) 22, no. 3: 619–631, at 628.
66a. Carl Peraino et al., *Cancer Research* (1971) 31: 1506–1512.
67. Robert Ader in *Environmental Variables in Animal Experimentation,* ed. Hulda Magalhaes (Lewisburg: Bucknell University Press, 1974) pp. 109–135, at 123.
68. Robert Ader, *Psychosomatic Medicine* (1967) 29, no. 4: 345–353.
69. R. Ader and S. B. Friedman, *Neuroendocrinology* (1968) 3: 378–386.
70. Alexander H. Freidman and Charles A. Walker, *Jrl. of Physiology* (1968) 197: 77–85.
71. M. P. Rogers et al., *Psychosomatic Medicine* (1979) 41, no. 2: 147–164 at 151.
72. Stanford B. Friedman et al., *Annals of the New York Academy of Sciences* (1969) 164: 381–393.
73. D. H. Sprunt and C. C. Flanigan, *Jrl. of Experimental Medicine* (1956) 104: 687–706. Cited by Stanford B. Friedman et al., ibid.
74. Robert Ader in *Environmental Variables in Animal Experimentation,* ed. Hulda Magalhaes (Lewisburg: Bucknell University Press, 1974) pp. 109–135, at 119–120.
74a. E. A. Emken, *Annual Review of Nutrition* (1984) 4: 339–376, at 365–367.
75. Morton Rothstein, *Biochemical Approaches to Aging* (New York: Academic Press, 1982) p. 258.
75a. S. Mitchell Harman et al., *Endocrinology* (1978) 102, no. 2: 540–544.
76. G. Miescher and C. Böhm, *Schweiz med. Wschr.* (1947) 77: 821–826. Cited by Annie M. Brown in *Animals for Research,* ed. W. Lane-Petter (New York: Academic Press, 1963) pp. 271 and 283.
76a. *Merck Index,* 10th ed. (Rahway, N.J.: Merck & Co., 1983) p. 3147.
77. John B. Jemmott, III et al., *Lancet* (June 25, 1983): 1400–1402.
78. Ziad Kronfol et al., *Life Sciences* (1983) 33: 241–247.
79. Stanley M. Bierman, *Western Jrl. of Medicine* (1983) 139, no. 4: 547–552.
80. Sharon Warren et al., *Jrl. of Chronic Diseases* (1982) 35: 821–831.
81. Stanislav V. Kasl et al., *Psychosomatic Medicine* (1979) 41, no. 6: 445–466.
82. Richard B. Shekelle et al., *Psychosomatic Medicine* (1981) 43, no. 2: 117–125.
83. Cary L. Cooper, *Jrl. of Human Stress* (1984) 10, no. 1: 4–11.
84. Steven Greer, *British Jrl. of Psychiatry* (1983) 143: 535–543.

85. Lawrence E. Hinkel, Jr. et al., *Psychosomatic Medicine* (1958) 20, no. 4: 278–295, at 295.
86. Richard H. Barnes et al., *Federation Proceedings* (1963) 22: 125–128.
87. Roman Kulwich et al., *Jrl. of Nutrition* (1953) 39: 639–645.
88. Richard H. Barnes et al., *Jrl. of Nutrition* (1957) 63: 489–498.
89. Richard H. Barnes and Grace Fiala, *Jrl. of Nutrition* (1958) 65: 103–114.
90. Richard H. Barnes et al., *Jrl. of Nutrition* (1959) 67: 599–610.
91. M. J. Sharkey, *Mammalia* (1971) 35: 162–168.
92. B. K. Armstrong and A. Softly, *British Jrl. of Nutrition* (1966) 20: 595–598.
92a. S. E. Olpin and C. J. Bates, *British Jrl. of Nutrition* (1982) 47: 577–588.
92b. R. J. Neale, *Laboratory Animals* (1984) 18: 119–124.
93. Frederick Hoelzel and Esther DaCosta, *Amer. Jrl. of Digestive Diseases* (1941) 8, no. 7: 266–270.
93a. Vernon Riley et al., *Cancer Detection and Prevention* (1979) 2, no. 2: 235–255.
93b. John K. Inglehart, *New England Jrl. of Medicine* (1985) 313, no. 6: 395–400.
93c. Thomas D. Overcast and Bruce D. Sales, *JAMA* (Oct. 11, 1985) 254, no. 14: 1944–1949.
94. Douglas K. Obeck, *Laboratory Animal Science* (1978) 28, no. 6: 698–704.
94a. Maxine Briggs in *Recent Vitamin Research*, ed. Michael H. Briggs (Boca Raton, Florida: CRC Press, 1984) p. 46.
95. M. W. Fox in *Environmental Variables in Animal Experimentation*, ed. Hulda Magalhaes (Lewisburg: Bucknell University Press, 1974) pp. 96–108, at 108.
95a. S. B. Friedman and R. Ader, *Neuroendocrinology* (1967) 2: 209–212.
95b. A. Wise and D. J. Gilburt, *Food and Cosmetic Toxicology* (1980) 18: 643–648.
95c. B. H. Ershoff, *American Jrl. of Clinical Nutrition* (1974) 27: 1395. Cited in ref. 95b.
95d. B. H. Ershoff, *Jrl. of Nutrition* (1977) 107: 822. Cited in ref. 95b.
95e. D. Kritchevsky, *Federation Proceedings* (1977) 36: 1692. Cited in ref. 95b.
95f. David M. Klurfeld et al., *Federation Proceedings* (March 5, 1986) 45, no. 4: 1076.
95g. Victor Herbert, *Science* (April 4, 1986) 232: 11.
95h. L. R. Jacobs, *Cancer Research* (1983) 43: 4057. Cited in ref. 95g.
95i. Hugh J. Freeman et al., *Cancer Research* (1980) 40: 2661–2665.
95j. Hugh J. Freeman in *Carcinogens and Mutagens in the Environment*, vol. 2, ed. Hans F. Stich (Boca Raton, Fla.: CRC Press, 1983) pp. 129–137, at 130.
95k. K. Wakabayashi et al., *Cancer Letters* (1978) 4: 171. Cited in ref. 95j.
95l. K. Watanabe et al., *Cancer Research* (1978) 38: 4427. Cited in ref. 95j.
96. R. A. Hinde, *Animal Behavior: A Synthesis of Ethology and Comparative Psychology*, 2nd ed. (New York: McGraw Hill, 1970.) Cited by S. Michael Plaut, *Pediatric Clinics of North America*, (1975) 22, no. 3: 619–631, at 620.
96a. Noel W. Solomons and Fernando E. Viteri in *Ascorbic Acid: Chemistry, Metabolism and Uses*, (Washington, D.C.: American Chemical Society, 1982) pp. 560–561.
97. S. A. Barnett, *Newsweek* (Dec. 3, 1973): 6–8. Cited by S. Michael Plaut, *Pediatric Clinics of North America* (1975) 22, no. 3: 619–631, at 621.
98. Panel on Non-human Primate Nutrition of the National Research Council of the National Academy of Sciences, *Nutrient Requirements of Nonhuman Primates* (Washington, D.C.: National Academy of Sciences, 1978).
99. Lowell A. Glasgow et al., *American Jrl. of Medicine* (July 20, 1982) 73, supp. 1A: 132–137.
99a. Mathew M. Ames et al., *Research Communications in Chemical Pathology and Pharmacology* (Oct., 1978) 22, no. 1: 175–185.
99b. John C. Bailar III, *New England Jrl. of Medicine* (Oct. 24, 1985) 313, no. 17: 1080–1081.
100. H. Babich, *Environmental Research* (1982) 29: 1–29, at 9.
100a. Elliot S. Vesell et al., *Federation Proceedings* (1976) 35: 1125–1132.
101. C. M. Brubaker et al., *Life Sciences* (1982) 30, no. 23: 1965–1971.

102. John B. Barnett, *International Archives of Allergy and Applied Immunology* (1981) 66: 229–232.
103. Carl J. Bodenstein, *Pediatrics* (1984) 73, no. 5: 733–736.
104. T. C. Chamberlin, *Jrl. of Geology* (1897) 5: 837–848. Cited by S. Michael Plaut, *Pediatric Clinics of North America* (1975) 22, no. 3: 619–631, at 628.

Chapter 1—220 References

1. Robert P. Heaney, *Jrl. of Laboratory and Clinical Medicine* (1982) 100: 309.
2. F. C. Redlich, *Jrl. of Medicine and Philosophy* (1976) 1, no. 1: 269–280.
3. Michael H. Kottow, *Medical Hypotheses* (1980) 6: 209–213.
4. George E. Vaillant, *New England Jrl. of Medicine* (1979) 301: 1249–1254.
5. S. Greer et al., *Lancet* (Oct. 13, 1979): 785–787.
5a. Keith W. Pettingale, Steven Greer et al., *Lancet* (March 30, 1985): 750.
6. J. Paget, *Surgical Pathology*, 2nd ed. (London: Longmans Green, 1870). Cited by S. Greer, *Psychological Medicine* (1979) 9: 81–89 at 82.
7. Lawrence LeShan, *Jrl. of the National Cancer Institute* (1959) 22, no. 1: 1–18.
8. Lawrence LeShan, *Annals of the New York Academy of Sciences* (1966) 125: 780–793.
9. Constance Holden, *Science* (1978) 200: 1363–1369.
10. Phillip Shaver et al., *American Jrl. of Psychiatry* (1980) 137, no. 12: 1563–1658.
11. Erik Agduhr, *Acta Medica Scandinavica* (1939) 99, no. 5: 387–424.
12. D. Drori and Y. Folman, *Experimental Gerontology* (1969) 4: 263.
13. D. Drori and Y. Folman, *Experimental Gerontology* (1976) 11: 25–32.
14. H. F. Smyth, Jr., *Food Cosmetic Toxicology* (1967) 5: 51–58.
15. Loren J. Chapman et al., *Jrl. of Abnormal Psychology* (1976) 85, no. 4: 374–382.
16. Martin Harrow et al., *American Jrl. of Psychiatry* (1977) 134, no. 7: 794–797.
17. Soon D. Koh et al., *Schizophrenia Bulletin* (1981) 7, no. 2: 292–307.
18. Mark Cook and Fredie Simukonda, *British Jrl. of Psychiatry* (1981) 139: 523–525.
19. Robert F. Simons, *Psychophysiology* (1982) 19, no. 4: 433–441.
20. Jan Fawcett et al., *Archives of General Psychiatry* (1983) 40: 79–84.
21. Robert H. D. Dworkin and Kathleen Saczynski, *Jrl. of Personality Assessment* (1984) 48, no. 6: 620–626.
22. Paul E. Meehl, *Bulletin of the Meninger Clinic* (1975) 39, no. 4: 295–307, at 299–300 and 305.
23. William S. Edell and Loren J. Chapman, *Jrl. of Consulting and Clinical Psychology* (1979) 47, no. 2: 379–384.
24. W. E. Penk et al., *Jrl. of Consulting and Clinical Psychology* (1979) 47, no. 6: 1046–1052.
25. Charles G. Watson, *Jrl. of Abnormal Psychology* (1972) 80, no. 1: 43–48.
25a. Charles G. Watson et al., *Psychological Reports* (1970) 26: 371–376.
26. E. Cuyler Hammond, *Jrl. of the National Cancer Institute* (May, 1964) 32: 1161–1188. Cited in *Wine of Life* by Harold J. Morowitz (New York: St. Martins Press, 1979).
27. Stephen L. Taylor, *New York Times* (Feb. 10, 1982).
28. Robert M. Nerem et al., *Science* (June 27, 1980) 208: 1475–1476.
28a. B. S. Gow, M. E. McCaskill and M. J. Legg, *Atherosclerosis* (1982) 44: 121–122.
28b. M. J. Legg, B. S. Gow and M. R. Roach, *Proc. Aust. Physiol. Pharmacol. Soc.* (1981) 12: 130 P. Cited in ref. 28a.
28c. S. Michael Plaut et al., *Psychosomatic Medicine* (1974) 36, no. 4: 311–320.
28d. S. Michael Plaut, *Developmental Psychology* (1970) 3, no. 3: 157–167.
29. W. B. Gross and Paul B. Siegel, *American Jrl. of Veterinary Research* (1982) 43, no. 11: 2010–2012.
30. W. B. Gross and P. B. Siegel, *American Jrl. of Veterinary Research* (1982) 43, no. 1: 137–139.
31. Jay R. Kaplan et al., *Arteriosclerosis* (1982) 2: 359–368.
32. John N. Edwards and David L. Klemmack, *Jrl. of Gerontology* (1973) 28, no. 4: 497–502.
33. Judith G. Rabkin and Elmer L. Struening, *Science* (1976) 194: 1013–1020.

34. Michael G. Marmot and S. Leonard Syme, *American Jrl. of Epidemiology* (1976) 104, no. 3: 225–247.
35. John G. Bruhn et al.,*Southern Medical Jrl.* (1982) 75, no. 5: 575–580, at 580.
36. Dianne Timbers Fairbank and Richard L. Hough,*Jrl. of Human Stress* (1979) 5: 41-47.
37. Jerry Suls et al., *Jrl. of Psychosomatic Research* (1979) 23: 315–319.
38. Irwin G. Sarason et al., *Psychosomatic Medicine* (1985) 47, no. 2: 156–163.
39. Rafaella M. A. Osti et al., *Psychotherapy and Psychosomatics* (1980) 33: 193–197.
39a. Carol W. Buck and Allan P. Donner, *Jrl. of Chronic Diseases* (1984) 37, no. 4: 247–253.
39b. T. Theorell, *Psychotherapy and Psychosomatics* (1980) 34: 135–148.
39c. D. G. Byrne, *British Jrl. of Medical Psychology* (1981) 54: 371–377.
39d. L. N. Gupta and R. K. Verma, *Indian Jrl. of Medical Research* (1983) 77: 697–701.
39e. Ralph Carasso, *International Jrl. of Neuroscience* (1981) 14: 223–225.
40. Thomas H. Holmes and Richard H. Rahe, *Jrl. of Psychosomatic Research* (1967) 11: 213–218.
41. Janice K. Kiecolt-Glaser et al., *Psychosomatic Medicine* (1984) 46, no. 1: 7–14.
42. Steven E. Locke et al., *Psychosomatic Medicine* (1984) 46, no. 5: 441–453.
42a. R. W. Bartrop et al., *Lancet* (April 16, 1977): 834–836.
42b. S. J. Schleifer et al., *JAMA* (1983) 250: 374–377.
42ba. Harold Levitan, *Psychosomatics* (Dec., 1985) 26, no. 12: 939–94.
42c. William A. Greene, *Jrl. of the American Medical Women's Assn.* (1965) 20, no. 2: 133–141, at 137.
42d. Knud J. Helsing et al., *American Jrl. of Public Health* (1981) 71, no. 8: 802–809.
43. W. P. Cleveland and D. T. Gianturco, *Jrl. of Gerontology* (1976) 31: 99–102. Cited in *Bereavement-Reactions, Consequences and Care*, ed. Marian Osterweis, Fredric Solomon and Morris Green (Washington, D.C.: National Academy Press, 1984).
43a. Guilia I. Perini et al., *Psychotherapy and Psychosomatics* (1984) 41: 48–52.
43b. Nancy A. Williams and Jerry L. Deffenbacher, *Jrl. of Human Stress* (1983) 9: 26–31.
43c. Barry Glassner and C. V. Halipur, *American Jrl. of Psychiatry* (1983) 140, no. 2: 215–217.
43d. G. H. B. Baker, *Psychotherapy and Psychosomatics* (1982) 38: 173–177.
43e. Richard Totman et al.,*Jrl. of Psychosomatic Research* (1980) 24: 155–163.
43f. Steven Lehrer, *Psychosomatic Medicine* (1980) 42, no. 5: 499–502.
43g. Francis Creed, *Lancet* (June 27, 1981): 1381–1385.
44. Kenneth B. Matheny and Penny Cupp, *Journal of Human Stress* (June, 1983): 14–23.
45. Paul J. Rosch, *JAMA* (1979) 242, no. 5: 427–428.
46. Hans Selye, *Stress and Distress* (New York: J. B. Lippincott, 1974).
46a. Rickey S. Miller and Herbert M. Lefcourt, *American Jrl. of Community Psychology* (1983) 11, no. 2: 127–139.
46b. W. D. Gentry et al., *Psychosomatic Medicine* (1982) 44: 195–202.
46c. Steven Greer and Maggie Watson, *Social Science and Medicine* (1985) 20, no. 8: 773–777.
46d. K. W. Pettingale et al., *Jrl. Psychsoc. Oncol.* In press. Cited in ref. 46c.
46e. L. Temoshok and B. H. Fox in *Impact of Psychoendocrine Systems in Cancer and Immunity*, ed. B. H. Fox and B. H. Newberry (New York: C. J. Hogrefe, 1984). Cited in ref. 46c.
46f. M. Watson et al., *Advances in the Biosciences, vol. 49—Psychological Aspects of Cancer*, ed. M. Watson and T. Morris (Oxford: Pergamon Press, 1984). Cited in ref. 46c.
46g. L. V. Holdeman et al., *Applied and Environmental Microbiology* (1976) 31, no. 3: 359–375.
46h. Marcia Angell, *New England Jrl. of Medicine* (1985) 312, no. 24: 1570–1572.
46i. Robert B. Case et al., *New England Jrl. of Medicine* (1985) 312, no. 12: 737–741.
47. Barrie R. Cassileth et al., *New England Jrl. of Medicine* (1985) 312, no. 24: 1551–1555.

47a. Austen Clark, in *Examining Holistic Medicine,* ed. Douglas Stalker and Clark Glymour (Buffalo, N.Y.: Prometheus Books, 1985) pp. 67–106.

47b. Edward R. Friedlander, in *Examining Holistic Medicine,* ibid., pp. 273–285.

48. Reubin Andres, *International Jrl. of Obesity* (1980) 4: 381–386.

49. A. R. Dyer et al., *Jrl. of Chronic Diseases* (1975) 28: 109–123. Cited by Ancel Keys in *Nutrition in the 1980's,* ed. Nancy Selvey and Philip L. White (New York: Alan R. Liss, 1981) pp. 31–46, at 39.

50. R. J. Garrison et al., *JAMA* (1983) 249: 2199–2203. Cited by Artemis P. Simopoulos, *Nutrition Reviews* (1985) 43, no. 2: 33–40.

50a. JoAnn E. Manson et al., *JAMA* (Jan. 16, 1987) 257, no. 3: 353-358.

50b. Ulf Smith, *Medical World News* (Feb. 11, 1985) 26, no. 3: 74.

51. Bernard Fisher et al., *New England Jrl. of Medicine* (1985) 312, no. 11: 665–673.

52. M. Alice Ottoboni, *The Dose Makes the Poison* (Berkeley, CA: Vincente Books, 1984) pp. 91–92.

53. Ibid., p. 94

54. *Federal Register* (Oct. 5, 1983) 48, no. 194: 45508.

55. W. W. Duke, *JAMA* (Nov. 6, 1915) 65, no. 19: 1600–1610.

56. Lawrence P. Garrod, *British Medical Jrl.* (Feb. 3, 1951): 205–210.

57. G. E. Foley and W. D. Winter, *Jrl. of Infectious Diseases* (1949) 85: 268. Cited by ref. 56.

58. T. D. Luckey, *Federation Proceedings* (Feb., 1978) 37, no. 2: 107–109.

58a. Committee to Study the Human Health Effects of Subtherapeutic Antibiotic Use in Animal Feeds, National Research Council, *The Effects on Human Health of Subtherapeutic Use of Antimicrobials in Animal Feeds* (Washington, D.C.: National Academy of Sciences, 1980) p. XIII.

58b. Ibid., p. 7

58c. Ibid., pp. 22–23.

58d. Scott D. Holmberg et al., *New England Jrl. of Medicine* (1984) 311, no. 10: 617–622.

58e. N. V. Medunitsyn, *Zh. Mikrobiol. Epidemiol. Immunobiol.* (1960) 31: 742–743.

59. Frank R. George et al., *Pharmacology, Biochemistry and Behavior* (1983) 19: 131–136.

60. Robert E. Hodges et al., *American Jrl. of Clinical Nutrition* (Aug., 1962) 11, no. 2: 85–93.

61. M. L. Smith and W. A. Loqman, *Archives of Andrology* (1982) 9: 105–113.

62. M. C. Chang, *Jrl. of Andrology* (1984) 5: 45-50.

63. C. Selli et al., *European Urology* (1983) 9: 109–112.

64. Robert T. Rubin et al., *Jrl. of Clinical Endocrinology and Metabolism* (1978) 47, no. 2: 447–452.

65. S. P. Ghosh et al., *Jrl. of Reproduction and Fertility* (1983) 67: 235–238.

66. P. Marrama et al., *Maturitas* (1982) 4: 131–138.

67. Herbert Y. Meltzer, *Jrl. of Pharmacology and Experimental Therapeutics* (1983) 224, no. 1: 21–27.

68. John T. Clark et al., *Science* (Aug. 24, 1984) 225–847–849.

69. Mark F. Schwartz et al., *Biological Psychiatry* (1982) 17, no. 8: 861–876.

70. A. Rocco et al., *Archives of Andrology* (1983) 10: 179–183.

71. L. C. Garcia Diez and J. M. Gonzalez Buitrago, *Archives of Andrology* (1982) 9: 311–317.

72. D. Ayalon et al., *Int. Jrl. of Gynaecology and Obstetrics* (1982) 20: 481–485.

72a. John Bancroft in *Biological Determinants of Sexual Behavior,* ed. J. B. Hutchison (New York: John Wiley & Sons, 1978) pp. 493–519, at 511.

72b. L. Lidberg, *Pharmakopopsychiat.* (1972) 5: 187. Cited in ref. 72a.

72c. L. Lidberg, *Hormones* (1972) 5: 273. Cited in ref. 72a.

72d. L. Lidberg and V. Sternthal, in prep. Cited in ref. 72a (p. 511).

73. Anon, *Science Digest* (July, 1982) 9: 94.

74. J. C. Theiss, *International Colloquium on Cancer*, Houston: M. D. Anderson Hospital and Tumor Institutes, 1981. Cited by*Lancet* (Dec. 11, 1982): 1317–1318.

75. Michael L. Kleinberg and Michael J. Quinn, *Amer. Jrl. Hosp. Pharm.* (1981) 38: 1301–1303.

76. Hanna Norppa et al., *Scand. Jrl. Work Envir. Health* (1980) 6: 299–301.

77. R. P. Bos, *Int. Arch. Occup. Environ. Health* (1982) 50: 359–369.

77a. Marja Sorsa et al., *Mutation Research* (1985) 154: 135–149.

78. S. Venitt et al.,*Lancet* (Jan. 14, 1984): 74–76.

79. *Lancet* (Dec. 11, 1982): 1317–1318.

80. J. F. Gibson et al., *Lancet* (Jan. 14, 1984): 100–101.

81. *Lancet* (Jan. 28, 1984): 203.

82. Luci A. Power and Michael H. Stolar,*Lancet* (March 10, 1984): 569–570.

82a. Sherry G. Selevan et al., *New England Jrl. of Medicine* (Nov. 7, 1985) 313, no. 19: 1173–1178.

82b. Eula Bingham,*New England Jrl. of Medicine* (Nov. 7, 1985) 313, no. 19: 1220–1221.

82c. Robert Hoover and Joseph F. Fraumeni, Jr., *Cancer* (1981) 47, no. 5: 1071–1080.

83. M. A. Firer et al., *British Medical Jrl.* (1981) 283: 693–696.

84. E. R. Stiehm et al., *Annals of Internal Medicine* (1982) 98: 80–93, cited by Richard D. de Shazo and John E. Salvaggio, *JAMA* (Oct. 26, 1984) 252, no. 16: 2198–2201.

84a. Gene P. Siegal et al., *Proceedings of the National Academy of Sciences* (1982) 79: 4064–4068.

85. Frederick Hoelzel and Esther DaCosta, *Amer. Jrl. of Digestive Diseases and Nutrition* (1937) 4: 325–331.

85a. James C. White, *New England Jrl. of Medicine* (1985) 312, no. 4: 246–247.

86. T. D. Luckey, *Health Physics* (1982) 43, no. 6: 771–789.

87. *Encyclopaedia Britannica*, 15th ed., vol. 15, "Radiation, Effects of" (Chicago: Encyclopaedia Britannica, 1979) pp. 378–392 at 386.

88. G. W. Beebe et al., cited by Alice M. Stewart, *Jrl. of Epidemiology and Community Health* (1982) 36: 80–86.

89. L. P. Breslavets et al., *Biophysics* (1960) 5, 86–87.

90. L. D. Carlson et al., *Radiation Research* (1957) 7: 190.

90a. Carolyn Ferree, *JAMA* (Dec. 6, 1985) 254, no. 21: 3036

91. Roy E. Albert et al.,*Radiation Research* (1961) 15: 410–430.

92. Wheeler P. Davey, *Jrl. of Experimental Zoology* (1919) 28, no. 2: 447–458.

93. T. D. Luckey, *Hormesis with Ionizing Radiation* (Boca Raton, Florida: CRC Press, 1980).

94. R. L. Sullivan and D. S. Grosch,*Nucleonics* (1953) 11: 21, cited by Luckey (ref. 93).

95. E. Lorenz et al., in *Biological Effects of External X and Gamma Radiation*, Part 1, ed. R. E. Zirkle (New York: McGraw Hill, 1954) p. 24, cited by Luckey (ref. 93).

96. J. J. Morris et al., *Effects of low level X radiation upon growth of mice*, unpublished report (1963), cited by Luckey (ref. 93).

97. L. P. Breslavets and A. S. Afanasyeva, *Vestn. Rentgenol. Radiol.* (1935) 14: 302 and *Cytologia* (1935) 8: 110, cited by Luckey, (ref. 93).

98. R. K. Schulz in *Survival of Food Crops and Livestock in the Event of Nuclear War*, ed. D. W. Benson and A. H. Sparrow (Oak Ridge, Tenn.: U.S. Atomic Energy Commission, 1971) p. 370, cited by Luckey (ref. 93).

99. I. Fendrik, *Stim. Newsletter* (1970) 1: 8, cited by Luckey (ref. 93).

100. A. S. Pressman, *Electromagnetic Fields and Life* (New York: Plenum Press, 1970) pp. 156–157.

101. C. M. Southam and J. Ehrlich,*Pythopathology* (1943) 33: 517–529.

102. T. D. Luckey in *Heavy Metal Toxicity, Safety and Hormology* by T. D. Luckey, B. Venugopal and D. Hutcheson (New York: Academic Press, 1975) p. 103.

103. House of Representatives no. 2284, 85th Congress, Second Session (1958).

103a. *Chicago Tribune* (June 28, 1985).

103b. Marjorie Sun, *Science* (1984) 223: 667–668.

103c. Marjorie Sun, *Science* (1985) 229: 739–741.

103d. David A. Kessler, *Science* (1984) 223: 1034–1040.

103e. W. Gary Flamm in *Carcinogens and Mutagens in the Environment,* vol. 1, ed. Hans F. Stich (Boca Raton, Florida: CRC Press, 1982) pp. 275–281.

104. Minna Alice Ottoboni, *The Dose Makes The Poison* (Berkeley, CA: Vincente Books, 1984) p. 99.

105. National Center for Toxicological Research, *Jrl. of Environmental Pathology and Toxicology* (1980) 3, no. 3. Cited in ref. 104.

106. Society of Toxicology Committee, *Fundamental and Applied Toxicology* (1981) 1, no. 1: 27–128. Cited in ref. 104.

107. *Physicians' Desk Reference,* 39th ed. (Oradell, N.J.: Medical Economics Co., 1985).

107a. David F. Horrobin, *Medical Hypotheses* (1981) 7: 115–125.

107b. *Physicians' Desk Reference,* 39th ed. (Oradell, N.J.: Medical Economics Co., 1985) pp. 1723–1724.

107c. Ibid., pp. 538 and 540.

107d. Ibid., p. 1051.

107e. Ibid., p. 532.

107f. Ibid., p. 1940.

107fa. *AMA Drug Evaluations,* 5th ed. (Chicago: American Medical Assn., 1983).

107fb. *Drug Facts and Comparisons* (St. Louis, Mo.: Facts and Comparisons, Inc., 1985).

107g. Joseph Meites et al., *Proceedings of the Society for Experimental Biology and Medicine* (1971) 137: 1225–1227.

107h. C. Huggins, *Cancer Research* (1965) 25: 1163. Cited in ref. 107g.

107i. R. I. Dorfman, *Methods in Hormone Research* (1965) 4: 165. Cited in ref. 107g.

107j. J. Hayward, *Recent Results in Cancer Research* (Berlin: Springer-Verlag, 1970) p. 69.

108. Mary E. Caldwell and Willis R. Brewer,*Cancer Research* (Dec., 1983) 43: 5775–5777.

108a. D. R. Stoltz et al., *Environmental Mutagenesis* (1984) 6: 343–354.

108b. S. Morris Kupchan and E. Bauerschmidt,*Photochemistry* (1971) 10: 664–666.

108c. Thomas S. Kuhn, *The Structure of Scientific Revolutions* (Chicago: University of Chicago Press, 1962) p. X.

108d. Ibid., p. 6.

108e. Ibid, p. 24.

108f. John Pfeiffer, *The Changing Universe* (New York: Random House, 1956) p. 142.

109. A. J. Clark, *The Mode of Action of Drugs on Cells* (London: Edward Arnold, 1933) cited by D. F. Horrobin,*Prostaglandins* (1977) 14, no. 4: 667–677.

110. E. J. Ariens et al., *Pharmacological Reviews* (1957) 9: 218–236.

111. J. M. Von Rossum in *Molecular Pharmacology,* vol. 2, ed. E. J. Ariens (New York: Academic Press, 1964) pp. 199–255. Do not confuse this book with the journal of the same name.

112. W. D. M. Paton, *Proc. of the Royal Society* (1961) 154B: 21–69.

112a. Richard N. Zare, *Science* (Oct. 19, 1984) 226: 298–303.

113. Seymour L. Romney et al., *Gynecologic Oncology* (1985) 20: 109–114.

114. Erhard Haus et al., *Science* (July 7, 1972) 177: 80–82.

115. F. Hallberg et al., *Experientia* (1973) 29, no. 8: 909–934.

116. L. E. Scheving et al., in *Chronobiology,* ed. Lawrence E. Scheving, Franz Halberg and John E. Pauly (Tokyo: Igaku Shoin Ltd., 1974) pp. 213–217.

117. Karel M. H. Philippens, in *Chronobiology,* ibid., pp. 23–28.

118. G. Brubacher et al.,*Bibliotheca Nutri, Dieta* (1981) 30: 90–99.

119. R. L. Gross and P. M. Newberne, *Physiological Reviews* (Jan., 1980) 60: 188–302, at 260.

119a. C. M. Leevy et al., *American Jrl. of Clinical Nutrition* (1965) 17: 259. Cited by ref. 119.

120. D. J. Smithard and M. J. S. Langman, *British Jrl. of Clinical Pharmacology* (1978) 5: 181–185.

120a. K. Bartlett, *Advances in Clinical Chemistry* (1983) 23: 141–198.

121. S. Harvey Mudd, *Jrl. of Clinical Pathology* 27 (Supplement *Royal College of Pathology,* 1974) 8: 38–47.

122. Charles Scriver, *Pediatrics* (1970) 36, no. 4: 493–496.

123. S. Harvey Mudd, *Advances in Nutritional Research,* vol. 4, ed. Harold H. Draper (New York: Plenum Pub., 1982) pp. 1-34.

124. E. Cheraskin and W. M. Ringsdorf, Jr., *New Hope for Incurable Diseases* (Jericho, N.Y.: Exposition, 1971).

124a. Noel S. Weiss, *New England Jrl. of Medicine* (Sept. 5, 1985) 313, no. 10: 632–633.

124b. Samuel M. Lesko et al., *New England Jrl. of Medicine* (1985) 313, no. 10: 593–596.

124c. Jon J. Michnovicz et al., *New England Jrl. of Medicine* (Nov. 20, 1986) 315, no. 21: 1305-1309.

124d. Cope, G. F., et al., *British Medical Jrl.* (Aug. 23, 1986) 291: 481.

124e. Roger Lewin, *Science* (Dec. 5, 1986) 234: 1200-1201.

125. Committee on Dietary Allowances of the Food and Nutrition Board, *Recommended Dietary Allowances,* 9th ed. (Washington, D.C.: National Academy of Sciences, 1980).

126. Eliot Marshall, *Science* (Oct. 25, 1985) 230: 420–421.

127. Henry Kamin, *Science* (Dec. 20, 1985) 230: 1324, 1326.

128. Robert E. Olson, *Science* (Dec. 20, 1985) 230: 1326.

129. Frank Press, *Science* (Dec. 20, 1985) 230: 1326, 1410.

130. Edward L. Schneider et al., *New England Jrl. of Medicine* (Jan. 16, 1986) 314, no. 3: 157–160.

131. Victor Herbert, *Federation Proceedings* (March 1, 1986) 45, no. 3: 477 (abstract no. 1885).

132. *Nutrition Today* (Nov./Dec., 1985): 4-23.

133. Food and Nutrition Board, *Jrl. of Nutrition* (1986) 116: 482–488.

134. Henry Kamin, *American Jrl. of Clinical Nutrition* (1985) 41: 165–170.

135. E. J. van der Beek, *Sports Medicine* (1985) 2: 175–197, at 179.

From page 326 of the BIG book. (Reference numbers refer to that book):

Possible Dangers of Simultaneously Administering Aspirin and Fish Oils

Aspirin and fish oils, as we have seen in Chapters 3 and 4, work through prostaglandin chemistry. Many of their benefits relate to thinning of the blood. The benefits are apparent but the dangers may be more subtle.

Hans Olaf Bang and Jorn Dyerberg[151] reported that, although Greenland Eskimos consume very little fish, they have a large intake of eicosapentenoic acid that derives from eating of whale and seals. Interestingly, the widely-held belief that the Greenland Eskimos have a low incidence of heart problems may be false. Claudi Galli cites M.C. Ehrström[152] as reporting that coronary heart disease in this population is quite common. (Greenland Eskimos also have nearly a 2-fold higher incidence of stroke than do their Danish counterparts.)[153] Attempting to draw dietary heart-health conclusions for fish eating, non-Eskimos from data relating to non-fish eating Eskimos who may have heart disease could be fraught with error.

Bang and Dyerberg[151] reported that "in four Greenland Eskimos with the longest bleeding time this measurement was repeated 24 hours after the intake of 1.5 grams acetylsalicylic acid." They found the bleeding times of the four Eskimos were shortened (rather than being lengthened as would normally be the case in non-takers of EPA). Thus the combination of aspirin and eicosapentenoic acid can result in a *reverse effect*.

George L. Royer et al.[154] relate that aspirin, and to a lesser extent ibuprofen (Motrin®), increase the values of serum glutamic oxaloacetic transaminase (SGOT), serum glutamic pyruvic transaminase (SGPT) and stool guaiac. Is it possible that fish oils (and other platelet deaggregators) might also detrimentally modify some of these same parameters? What other dangers may exist in the consumption of fish oils, especially if complicated by simultaneously taking aspirin, tetracycline, quinidine, quinine, heparin, protamine sulphate, warfarin (Coumadin®) or other anticoagulant, antiaggregating drugs, vitamins and foods?

How to Give a Gift or Memorial to Your Local Library, and to Libraries of Nearby Colleges and Universities Including your Alma Mater

Here's an idea for persons who wish to add an appropriate "personalized" touch to their giving—as an individual or as a group. A gift of Walter A. Heiby's *The Reverse Effect: How Vitamins and Minerals Promote Health and CAUSE Disease* reflects the taste of the giver or, in the case of memorials, of the individual in whose memory it is given. Moreover, such a gift provides an excellent way for a health-minded organization to help the community. A gift book may also be given in the name of your daughter, son, parent, or other relative in commemoration of a special occasion (e.g., high school or college graduation, birthday, anniversary). A book donation also makes an excellent Christmas or "thank-you" present. (The honored person will point with pride to this book in the library and to the inscription honoring him or her.) A library can use more than one copy of this book should you desire to honor more than one person.

Suggestion: Send your community newspaper a notice of your gift, preferably with a photograph of the person being honored and/or your photo. Perhaps your newspaper would prefer to photograph you making the presentation to the librarian.

Simply write out or send this form to each library:

I would like to establish a gift or memorial. I hearby donate the enclosed sum of $59.50 for the purchase of *The Reverse Effect: How Vitamins and Minerals Promote Health and CAUSE Disease* by Walter A. Heiby (published by: MediScience Publishers, P.O. Box 256-P, Deerfield, IL 60015), ISBN 0-938869-01-9.

Please inscribe the inside front cover of this book to show it is a:

☐ gift from the undersigned
☐ memorial in the honor of _____
                                (Name of person honored)
☐ gift in the honor of _____
                                (Name of person honored)

I would like an acknowledgment sent to:

_____
(Relative or friend's name)

_____
(Address)

Signed:_____

Address:_____

City:_____State:_____Zip:_____

If you decide against using this form show it to your librarian anyway. Your library might like to adapt it for use in soliciting donations for other books.

"When I get a little money, I buy books; and if
any is left, I buy food and clothes."
—Desiderius Erasmus

"A good book, in the language of the book-
sellers, is a salable one; in that of the curious,
a scarce one; in that of men of sense, a useful
and instructive one."
—Talbot Wilson Chambers

"The books that help you most are those that
make you think the most."
—Theodore Parker

"The best of a book is not the thought which it
contains, but the thought which it suggests; just
as the charm of music dwells not in the tones but
in the echoes of our hearts."
—Oliver Wendell Holmes

"It is one of the more fascinating aspects of the
history of science that you could actually make a
list of inventions which, if they had been made
correctly too early, would have brought science
to a standstill. Let me give you a simple
example. If Mendeleev had known where to place
helium—which was already a known gas by the
time that he made the periodic table—the whole
table would have been out of kilter. Because he
would have had to ask, where are the other gases?
Where is argon, krypton, and that whole line of
gases?"
—Jacob Bronowski, A Sense of the Future
(Cambridge, Mass: The MIT Press, 1977) p.
231.

"....the highlights of tomorrow are the
unpredictabilities of today."
—Cesar Milstein, Science (March 14, 1986) 231:
1261-1268 at 1267.

Every progressive spirit is opposed by a
thousand men appointed to guard the past."
—Maurice Maeterlinck, The Bluebird.

ORDER FORM

MediScience Publishers
PO Box 256-P
Deerfield, IL 60015

Consider the Big Book and the sampler as gifts for scientific and health-minded friends. Why not make your colleagues aware of the *reverse effect* by giving or sending each of them the sampler?

Enclosed is my check or money order (checks on U.S. banks or international money order in U.S. funds if a foreign order) for which please send the following books by Walter A. Heiby. (Sorry, but we cannot accept open account or C.O.D. orders.)

Quantity	Book	Exten.
	Better Health and the Reverse Effect (ISBN 0-938869-03-5). A sampler containing "How to Read Biomedical Literature" and "How to Use the *Reverse Effect* and the *Pleasure Concept*" as well as the associated reference lists from *The Reverse Effect: How Vitamins and Minerals Promote Health and CAUSE Disease.* For use as an introduction to the *reverse effect* and for the guidance of laboratory scientists in designing biomedical experiments. Paperback, each $3.95 ($.26), 4-9 copies, each $3.75 ($.24), 10-99 copies, each $3.50 ($.23), 100 or more, each $3.25 ($.21). *	
	The Reverse Effect: How Vitamins and Minerals Promote Health and CAUSE Disease (ISBN 0-938869-01-9). The First Edition of the big 1216-page volume, cloth bound and Smythe sewn, using acid-free paper to stay white for centuries. Each $59.50 ($3.87); 2-4 copies, each $54.50 ($3.54); 5-9 copies, each $52.50 ($3.41); 10 or more, each $49.50 ($3.22).*	

* All prices postpaid at book rate to USA destinations. Amounts shown in parentheses are sales taxes per book if shipped to an Illinois address. Foreign customers: Please add $2.00 for each sampler ($1.00 each for 10 or more) and $8 for each big book for delivery by surface mail.

Subtotal_____

6 1/2% sales tax (if Ill.)_____

Foreign Postage_____

Total enclosed_____

I understand orders not subject to a quantity discount may be returned for prompt refund. (No return privilege on quantity-discount orders or on foreign orders unless damaged or defective when you receive them.)

Name:_____

Company or Institution:_____

Address:_____

City:_____State:_____Zip:_____

Book Investors: The First Edition of the big book, if ordered in lots of ten or more copies will be autographed by the author, on request, for possible additional value as a long-term investment. Check here if 10 or more copies of the big book are being ordered and autographs are desired☐.

From page 260 of the BIG book. (Reference numbers refer to that book):

Hypothesis:
A *Reverse Effect* Involving Aspirin and Cancer Metastases Will Be Discovered.

We have seen that the work of James J. Kolenick et al.[264] and of Gabriel Gasic et al.[265] showed aspirin inhibits formation of metastases in cancerous mice. We also observed that the *in vitro* research of Duff and Duran[241d] found that the T-cell proliferative response to interleukin-2 was increased at 39° C (i.e., under fever conditions) compared to 37° C. Recently, Steven A. Rosenberg et al.,[310] Beverly Merz,[311] Michael T. Lotze et al.[312] and Charles G. Moertel,[313] as well as subsequent studies published in the *New England Jrl. of Medicine* of April 9, 1987, reported that metastatic cancer was favorably treatable with interleukin-2. Interleukin-2 not only activates helper and cytotoxic T-cells but also that special kind of lymphocyte, the natural killer cell.

Putting these facts in juxtaposition suggests that aspirin, through its fever-lowering power, will tend to inhibit the T-cell proliferative response to interleukin-2, thereby reducing the T-cell's cancer combatting potential and thus cancer metastases might be promoted. But the studies of Kolenick and of Gasic indicate, to the contrary, that aspirin can reduce the formation of metastases. We can therefore speculate that at some dosage aspirin's power to lower fever and thereby to reduce the action of the T-cell proliferative response (i.e., aspirin's possible tendency to *increase* metastases) will be overcome by aspirin's power to *reduce* metastases. At that dosage level there should occur a *reverse effect* in aspirin's influence on metastases. Determining dosage levels at which *reverse effects* occur, not only with aspirin but with various other drugs in different disease states, could be important in optimizing therapies.
